good food
for life

good food for life

PLANNING, PREPARING, AND SHARING

Maggie Davis
MS, RD, LDN, FADA, CDE

PARACLETE PRESS
BREWSTER, MASSACHUSETTS

Good Food for Life: Planning, Preparing, Sharing

2010 First Printing

ISBN: 978-1-55725-627-0

Library of Congress Cataloging-in-Publication Data
Davis, Maggie, 1975-
  Good food for life : planning, preparing, sharing / Maggie Davis.
      p. cm.
  Includes index.
  ISBN 978-1-55725-627-0
  1. Nutrition. I. Title.
  RA784.D385 2010
  613.2--dc22   2010018454

10 9 8 7 6 5 4 3 2 1

Published by Paraclete Press
Brewster, Massachusetts
www.paracletepress.com
Printed in the United States of America

Contents

Foreword

HAVE YOU EVER SAT IN A NUTRITIONIST'S WAITING ROOM? There are lovely flowers on a table in the corner, a pleasant receptionist typing away at the desk, and a variety of lifestyle magazines on the coffee table. Now, imagine that you are the founder of a Christian weight-loss program that has reached over a million people. Why would she be there? Surely she would already know all that needs to be known about such things! Surely she'd only be there to have a business meeting of some kind.

Well, I am that founder, and I was uncomfortable before my first meeting with Maggie Davis, MS, RD, LDN, FADA, CDE, the author of the book you are holding in your hand. We all need nutritional wisdom, including me! I went to see Maggie for advice for my own life. Meeting her became a turning point in nearly every area of my life—transforming my relationship with food and with God.

What I love most about Maggie is that she isn't about making people thin. She's not about diet as something we do to make us thin. Instead, she's about wellness and nutrition and education. That first meeting was the beginning of an important friendship. We now work together to help people see their whole life as interconnected—body, soul, and spirit.

Two years ago, Maggie and I co-authored a book entitled *Your Whole Life: The 3D Plan for Eating Right, Living Well, and Loving God.* The program I had developed thirty-five years earlier was completely revamped for a new generation of women and men. A generation ago, I used to talk about what I called the three "Ds"—diet, discipline, and discipleship. But more recently, I updated that language to be more useful to women and men today. So Maggie and I focused ourselves (I'm the plan's first and most devoted member!) and others on eating right, living well, and loving God.

Good Food for Life: Planning, Preparing, and Sharing is full of wisdom and fun. It builds upon what we did together in *Your Whole Life.* You will love every page of it, and you'll learn much about the beauty of food and what things you can do with food that will enrich your life. All too many of us, because of weight issues, have come to see food as the enemy: something to avoid, something to eat as little as possible, something we dread even thinking about. The end result of these negative thoughts is that we don't plan or enjoy the preparation of good meals, and we end up eating the wrong foods, running through mealtime, and snacking with all the wrong things at the wrong time. With Maggie in your corner, you'll learn that food is a pleasure, not something to fear.

I have been in Maggie's home. She's a gourmet cook, entertains beautifully, and absolutely loves food and its presentation. I promise you that if you follow her example and begin to look at the colors on your plate, if you begin to plan your meals and shop a little differently, if you try a whole grain, or if you even read a label or two a week, your health will change, and not only will you lose a little weight, but you'll gain a lot of insight, too.

Maggie will walk you through your kitchen, look on your shelves, and check the refrigerator. She'll take you to the grocery store, show you how to read labels, and tell you what you should plant out back, if possible. What fun is in store for you within the pages of this book! Food and nutrition will look a lot different to you after you read *Good Food for Life*.

The story of the Garden of Eden is one in which you'll see how God used food to teach us the biggest lessons of life. Do we listen to God? Do we listen to our own desires? Then, at the end of the Bible, God talks about a banquet table where we will all gather to celebrate his love. And in between the beginning and the end of the Bible there's manna from heaven, loaves and fishes, water and wine, and many other stories centered around food. It's interesting that God used food so often to teach his people about love, family, fun, faith, and trust. Let's do the same.

With all my heart I endorse this book, and I thank God for Maggie and her work in my life.

Carol Showalter

Carol D. Showalter
www.3DYourWholeLife.com

Introduction

The ordinary acts we practice every day at home are of more importance to the soul than their simplicity might suggest.
—Thomas Moore, *Care of the Soul,* 1994

RE YOU READY TO ENJOY HEALTHIER FOOD and to live well every day? Do you want to know more about which foods are healthy, how to plan your meals, and how get the most from the food you buy?

Good Food for Life follows alongside *Your Whole Life: The 3D Plan for Eating Right, Living Well, and Loving God,* which Carol Showalter wrote in 2007 to capture more than three decades of experience in living a healthy, whole Christian lifestyle. I was thrilled when Carol asked me to contribute the nutrition advice and information to that book, and I'm thrilled now to be sharing my expertise in "good food" with readers who have followed the 3D Plan and with those who are new to the concept. Think of this book as your road map for eating better for your whole life—one day at a time, one meal or snack at a time. I invite you to join me on a journey to transform your food habits and to live well. You will learn not only what to eat, but also how to manage daily meals, and how to share your table with others in ways that bring beauty into your life.

In a world that is as full of diet books as it is of rich and overfilling foods, *Good Food for Life* offers you the important middle ground—ways to make healthy eating part of your everyday life as well as an ingredient in the feasts you celebrate. This book is part information, part inspiration, part art, and part science.

In a world that is as full of diet books as it is of rich and overfilling foods, Good Food for Life offers you the important middle ground.

Together we'll explore aspects of food and nutrition in a practical way to inform and to inspire you to improve your daily life. This volume is more than a compilation of menus and recipes. It offers an approach to managing meals, snacks, and splurges—and takes you from planning to food presentation at the table. This book is your resource for making meals a nourishing, enjoyable, and sacred part of your day. It is a tool that can help you to simplify and improve your everyday life in unexpected ways by applying personal values to your daily habits. Making good food a priority can help to nourish us and reduce the household food budget, lessen the burden on our planet, and better achieve our higher goals in life.

We all love programs and diets, don't we? We love to feel that—with each new plan—we can turn our lives around. And sometimes it actually happens; but most often, again and again, people all but overdose on diets and strict plans without ever making real changes in their habits. There must be a better way. In 1975, Carol Showalter sought a better way and developed 3D, a faith-based diet program, to meet her own needs as well as the needs of other women in her church, where her husband was the pastor. For thirty-five years, this plan has helped over a million people change their lives by focusing every day on eating right, living well, and loving God. Since *Your Whole Life* was published in 2007, Carol and I have been speaking to groups representing the full spectrum of Christian denominations about this mind, body, and spirit approach. We have received an enthusiastic response from audiences and from those who are actively involved in 3D groups in their workplace or church. This book was written to provide even more detail about eating right and practical advice about applying the 3D principles in daily life.

To consume good food as part of a healthy lifestyle takes time and tailoring to the individual or the family. One reason many diet programs don't work beyond the first few weeks is that they impose a particular way of eating, a narrow range of food choices, and very specific menus without teaching the reader the principles of selecting and enjoying a wide variety of foods. That's why I work with clients to help make changes that are likely to last a lifetime. So, no, I cannot promise you a miracle when you read this book, prepare the recipes, and serve the menus that you find here. But I can challenge you to a new way of thinking. I can challenge you to do the work and share the joys and hardships that come with achieving any worthwhile goal.

Diet books give us rules and menus that tell us what we should eat for a certain period of time, from days or weeks to several months. The implied promise is that if you are able to eat this exact menu for a certain period of time you will lose weight—keep exactly to the diet, they intimate, or you won't lose weight. But this book asks you to get involved in the process of creating healthful meals with thought and consideration, from beginning to end. To eat right and enjoy good food for your whole life, you will need to rethink your approach to food. I have never worked with an individual or a family who could rely solely on a one-size-fits-all menu for all its needs. And I have never worked with anyone who could survive on prepackaged food plans or liquid meal replacements for any extended period of time. What most of us need are plans tailored to the way we work and live our lives.

Good Food for Life is designed to help you find easy ways to eat right for your whole life, one day at a time, one meal or one snack at a time. The transformation begins long before you go grocery shopping or turn on the stove, so we will explore simple and easy ideas for planning meals and selecting recipes that you will enjoy preparing and eating. Then we'll look at ways to get your kitchen in good working order—good food is much easier to prepare when your kitchen environment is organized and user-friendly.

Good Food for Life is designed to help you find easy ways to eat right for your whole life, one day at a time, one meal or one snack at a time.

Once the planning's done we'll venture out to shop for food and examine the options that might work best for your budget, your available time, and your personal health goals. We'll look at efficient ways to store your food to preserve its quality and to get the most out of the items you've purchased. And you will find simple techniques for preparing food in advance, as well as for seasoning foods with simple herbs and spices even if you don't have time to follow a detailed recipe. Good taste and good health should not be mutually exclusive concepts! We'll explore techniques to achieve both of these important goals.

In *Good Food for Life* you will also find advice on using daily good food targets and learn how to apply these guidelines to your own particular needs. The book includes sample menus to show how you can eat the recommended types of foods in actual meals and snacks in a variety of different ways. These samples can also be an effective tool for creating your own daily menus. The sample menus will also prompt you to include adequate portions of fruits and vegetables into your day. Along with these menus you'll have tools to evaluate the food you buy and eat: the nutrition facts label and online-based sources of information.

In the Sharing section of this book, you will see how you can combine eating right with living well. Good food involves so much more than just what you eat. Making a commitment to keep your mealtimes sacred is equally important. If you pay attention to the

> If you pay attention to the where, when, and how of eating you can take your diet— your usual meals and snacks— from good to great.

where, when, and how of eating you can take your diet—your usual meals and snacks—from good to great. For example, make lunch a time to refuel your mind, body, and spirit by mindfully focusing on the food as you relax and eat. You'll go back to work feeling satisfied and refreshed.

Eating meals that you yourself have prepared is perhaps the easiest and least expensive way to enjoy good food, but eating out is frequently a necessary part of our lives as we travel or manage busy schedules, so I will give you tips for making informed choices. And beyond just dining out, I have also included a sample buffet menu and recipes that would be suitable for any celebration or holiday get-together.

I have compiled a week of menus for each of the four seasons of the year, which are typical of the type of meals that you can plan for yourself and your household. And I have included recipes for foods that are featured in the menus so that you can try some of them and refer to them when looking at recipes from other sources. I have also given examples of what you can select for your "choice calories" and even some examples of splurges included in a particular menu. And I will give you easy tools to evaluate the food you eat—using the nutrition facts label and online sources of information.

As you read this book you will want to decide what areas need attention first. You may have a good knowledge of nutrition but not have much cooking skill. Or you may be a gourmet cook but travel on business and need to learn to make better restaurant choices. I will give you ideas for managing these situations. You may be a skilled gourmet cook but not be aware of how to make the food you cook be more nutritious by including more vegetables in your menus or by substituting whole grains for refined ones. Or you may realize that you arrive home every evening and feel stressed by deciding what to eat when you're ravenously hungry. Simply planning the night before can decrease your stress and increase the likelihood of having good food for dinner.

You don't have to change everything at once. You just need to decide where to start, and that starting point will be different for each of you.

I have included stories and experiences of some of my clients and patients, but I have changed the names to protect their privacy.

Now, before we go into the kitchen and get started, let's just briefly review some important nutrition facts that we'll use when we're planning what to eat!

● ● ● ● ● ● ● ● ● ● ● ●　P L A N N I N G

Nutrition Basics

If more of us valued food and cheer and song
above hoarded gold, it would be a merrier world.
—J.R.R. Tolkien (1892–1973)

GOOD FOOD FOR LIFE IS A PRACTICAL GUIDEBOOK to help you include good food in your daily diet. I don't use the term *diet* in the sense of a restrictive way of eating, but rather as a word that describes the foods you usually eat. Whether you're trying to lose weight, gain weight, or maintain a healthy weight, you'll benefit from consuming a variety of healthy foods in moderation and balancing your intake day to day. Now let's go over some basic nutrition information before we explore the planning, preparing, and sharing aspects of good food.

First, there is no one perfect meal plan or menu or calorie level that is right for everyone. The human body can be sustained on a wide variety of foods if the energy in the food we eat is equal to the energy we burn. In times of famine the body can adapt to having less than usual. Individuals who have gone on hunger strikes can survive for weeks without eating solid food. Our bodies are designed to tap into our stores of fat, protein in our muscles and organs, and minerals and vitamins stored in our bones and other body tissues. But in daily life we strive not merely for survival but for optimum health. The best way to move toward healthful living is to provide our body with the daily nourishment of good foods in appropriate amounts for each of us.

The advice offered in this book is based on current nutrition research, in other words, what the best scientific evidence available teaches us at the present time. Of course we need to stay tuned for new information, because the work being done in genetic research is likely to make us more aware of our actual individual needs in the years to come.

> The human body can be sustained on a wide variety of foods if the energy in the food we eat is equal to the energy we burn.

In reviewing individual diet histories with elderly nursing home residents, I have seen a wide variety of cultures and ethnic backgrounds—all of which speak specifically to eating preferences. Some of these elders have always eaten well, and others have always eaten whatever was available or only what they liked. Most of my clients are somewhere in the middle. What they ate as growing children and young adults may hold important clues to their longevity, in addition to their genetic legacy. But I have seen that learning about what constitutes good healthy food can lead to eating right and to decreased risk of chronic diseases and better control of chronic conditions such as diabetes and heart disease.

Today we are bombarded in all types of media with capsule news of the latest nutrition and medical research results. Bulletins are often sound bites that oversimplify or exaggerate study results. You see headlines about the "ten best foods to prevent cancer" or "miracle fruits" or "bad carbs." So how do you know what to eat and how much? You don't have to become a registered dietitian or licensed nutritionist to select good foods. But you do want to begin with the basics, so here are some frequently asked questions with guidance for nutrition and basic approaches to foods and thoughtful eating practices.

what good foods do we need TO INCLUDE IN OUR EVERYDAY DIET ?

ALTHOUGH CALORIES ARE OFTEN WHAT COME TO MIND when individuals are trying to eat better and care for their well-being, how we distribute those calories among good foods is perhaps even more important. We need a variety of fruits, vegetables, whole grains, lean protein, and healthy fats. The following chart will help you to figure out what number of portions would be an ideal amount of each good food to try to include each day. You will find typical portions of these types of foods in Appendix B (Food Groups: Serving Size Comparisons).

For women and those over 55, about 1600 Calories' worth of servings of the core foods is a good target each day. For men or very active women, the 2200-Calorie level would be a reasonable target, and for active men the 2800-Calorie level. You can see that if your food intake is in the 2000-Calorie range (the number of Calories that are used for a guideline on the Nutrition Facts labels that we will look at in chapter 5), you should consider eating 3 fruits each day and at least 6 servings per day of vegetables.

Now, that doesn't mean that you need to eat 6 different vegetables. For example, if you have a spinach salad for lunch that has 3 cups of raw spinach, mushrooms, and onions (3 servings), and 2 stalks of celery with peanut butter (1 serving) for a snack, and 1 cup of green beans (2 servings) for dinner, you would have had a total of 6 servings of vegetables that day.

The following chart gives some specific good food targets to include in your daily meal plan based on how many calories you need. The more food your body needs, the more fruits, vegetables, and other good foods you can eat. These targets can help you compare what types of foods and the portions you usually are eating and let you know what you could eat more of or less of to be as healthy as you can be. This doesn't mean you need to sit down and count calories. And a word of caution: do not cut your calorie intake below the 1200-Calorie level without the advice of your registered dietitian, certified diabetes educator, or physician.

good food targets VARY WITH THE AMOUNT OF FOOD YOU EAT

RECOMMENDED SERVINGS OF THESE CORE FOODS provide a balance of the major nutrients: carbohydrates, protein, and fat. (For recommended serving sizes, see Appendix B.) These nutrients are the major source of the fuel (calories) that our bodies and brains need to survive and to repair our cells. For infants, children, and pregnant and lactating women, these nutrients are also necessary for growth as well as repair.

To determine how many calories
you specifically need each day, go to
www.3DYourWholeLife.com/goodfood
to calculate your specific needs.
This method asks you enter your usual activity level to
determine your own unique needs. And don't forget to
recalculate the calories if you have a significant change in
your weight or your exercise level, since these factors will
change the amount of fuel your body needs.

Recommended Daily Portion Guidelines

food group	calories/ serving	800	1000	1200	1400
Vegetables	25	3	3	4	4
Fruits	80	2	2	2	2
Whole Grains	80	2	3	3	3
Starches (1 oz)	80	0	0	0	1
High Calcium Foods	100	1.5	1.5	2	2
Lean High Protein Foods	35–75	4	4	5	6
Oils & Other Fats	50	1	2	3	4
Water/ no-cal drinks (8 oz)	0	5	5	6	6

		800	1000	1200	1400
Core Food Calories		750	900	1050	1250
Your Choice Calories		50	100	150	150
Total Calories		800	1000	1200	1400

what foods do we need to eat less often OR ELIMINATE FROM OUR MEALS AND SNACKS?

MINIMIZE FOODS THAT CONTAIN ADDED SUGARS, saturated fats, trans fats, cholesterol, salt, or sodium, and minimize the amount of alcohol you drink (no more than 1 alcoholic beverage per day for women, 2 or fewer per day for men). And reduce your intake of processed and refined foods as much as possible. It's also important to know that salty, fatty, and sugary foods are appetite-enhancers, and they may begin to stimulate your hunger with the first bite. Saturated fats can also decrease your body's ability to know when you've had enough to eat.

1600	1800	2000	2200	2400	2600	2800	3000
5	6	6	6	7	7	8	8
3	3	3	3	3	3	4	4
3	3	4	4	5	5	6	6
2	3	3	4	4	5	5	6
2	3	3	3	3	3	3	3
6	6	6	7	7	7	8	8
5	5	6	7	7	8	9	10
7	7	8	8	9	9	10	10

1450	1650	1825	2000	2100	2300	2450	2600
150	150	175	200	300	300	350	400
2600	1800	2000	2200	2400	2600	2800	3000

how do you define A HEALTHY DIET?

A HEALTHY DIET CAN TAKE MANY FORMS, but it should include a variety of carbohydrates, protein, and fat; water; and vitamins, minerals, and antioxidants found in real food. A healthy diet contains foods that are prepared and stored safely, minimizing the chance of food poisoning. And a healthy diet should meet the needs of the individual eating it, depending on medical condition, age, exercise level, and any other factors that may affect metabolic needs, such as pregnancy or chemotherapy. A healthy diet should also be designed to meet the food budget of the individual or household.

how often SHOULD YOU EAT?

SOME FOLKS CAN'T EAT THEIR FIRST MEAL BEFORE 10 AM while others feel hungry as soon as they wake up in the early morning. It's still the total calories that count the most, but how you distribute the fuel to your body may make a difference. Research shows that individuals who eat four to six times per day are the most successful in maintaining a healthy weight. And eating more often can help prevent extreme hunger, which can lead to overeating at the next meal. Try to not go more than 4 to 5 hours between meals and snacks to keep your body evenly fueled and keep hunger under control. Eating smaller meals more often can also be helpful in stabilizing blood sugar levels in those individuals with diabetes or with low blood sugar.

what are the current recommendations regarding CALORIES, SODIUM INTAKE, FAT, ADDED SUGARS, MICRONUTRIENTS SUCH AS VITAMINS, MINERALS, AND ANTIOXIDANTS, AND SO ON?

FOLLOWING ARE SOME OF THE GENERAL GUIDELINES for specific nutrient intake. Keep in mind that new research evidence is being published so frequently that recommendations may change that would override the advice listed below in the future. These guidelines may vary with an individual's medical condition and may need to be adjusted with consultation by your registered dietitian. To find a Registered Dietitian in your area, ask your doctor for a recommendation or visit the American Dietetic Association's website at www.eatright.org and click on "Find a Registered Dietitian."

■ calories Americans actually consume nearly 3800 Calories per day if we average the intake of all U.S. adults regardless of their needs. By now you should have a target calorie range using one of the methods listed above. Some days you may consume more or less than other days, but think of your target calorie range as an average intake over the course of a week. Balancing your intake of good food with exercise is an important part of managing your weight and keeping your body healthy. If you are consuming more food than you need right now, consider decreasing your meals and snacks slowly, allowing your body to adjust and your mind and spirit to get used to the changes. Never cut more than 500 Calories a day without advice from your healthcare provider.

■ sodium — The average person in the United States consumes about 3000 to 4500 mg of sodium each day, and yet our bodies need only a minimum of 250 mg of sodium daily. One quarter of a teaspoon of table salt contains about 500 mg. Sea salt contains just as much sodium as mined table salt. Many processed foods contain over 1000 mg per serving. Restaurant entrees may contain over 2000 mg. Good food containing less than 2300 mg per day is recommended for healthy individuals; less than 1500 mg daily is best for those with hypertension or who are salt-sensitive, middle-aged or older adults, or African Americans.

■ potassium — The daily recommendation for potassium is 4700 mg per day, which is about double the amount of sodium needed per day. Major sources are fruits and vegetables, so meeting the daily portion guidelines for these foods will insure that you get enough. Individuals on certain medications such as diuretics, which cause you to lose potassium, may need to eat more high-potassium foods. If you have certain medical conditions such as kidney failure, you may be advised by your healthcare provider to limit potassium to a specific level. A nutrition professional can help you to customize your meals and snacks.

■ carbohydrates — Try to consume at least 3 servings of whole grains. Half or more of all the grains you eat in a day should be whole grains. The more calories you burn each day, the more carbohydrates you will need. Try substituting whole-grain flour or white whole-wheat flour for ¼ of the white flour in a recipe. And look for whole-grain cereals that are minimally processed, such as shredded wheat or old-fashioned (steel cut) oatmeal. These foods will be metabolized more slowly than cereals that are more processed or refined and will keep you full longer after eating them. Whole grains will also contain all of the vitamins and minerals that occur naturally in the grain, not just the nutrients that have been put back in the enrichment process.

■ fiber — Most adults need somewhere between 20 and 40 grams of fiber each day. The higher your calorie intake, the higher your fiber intake should be. Increase your fiber intake gradually so that your digestive system can adjust. Eating more fruits, vegetables, and whole grains will insure that your fiber intake is in the healthy range.

■ added sugars The most specific guideline for limiting added sugar intake was issued by the American Heart Association in August 2009 (www.AmericanHeart .org). These recommendations advise that women consume no more than 100 Calories (less than 6 teaspoons or 24 grams) per day of added sugar and that men consume no more than 150 Calories (less than 9 teaspoons or 36 grams) per day of added sugar. Most Americans now consume more than 360 Calories (22 teaspoons or 90 grams) of sugar per day. Even individuals with diabetes can plan small amounts of sugar into their meals and snacks. Be aware that sugar added to foods may be listed by other names in the ingredient list on packaged foods (such as glucose, fructose, dextrose, corn syrup, agave syrup, honey, brown rice syrup, malt and many others). The bottom line is to keep your added sugar intake as low as possible most days.

■ fat A moderate fat intake, similar to the Mediterranean diet, rather than a very low fat intake may be healthiest for most individuals. The Mediterranean diet includes less saturated fat (for example, animal fats and hydrogenated fats such as shortening) but more monounsaturated fats and omega-3s from fish, nuts, olives, and olive oil than the typical American diet. There is some evidence that intake of the omega-3s called EPA and/or DHA from fish or omega-3 fish oil supplements may help decrease the risk of diabetes, macular degeneration, and prostate cancer. It may also decrease the risk of fatal heart attacks in those individuals who have heart disease. Don't take more than 1000 mg per day without consulting with your Registered Dietitian or health care provider. Fat is necessary for our overall health and to provide the satisfaction we look for after eating. You can visit the American Heart Association website at www.myfatstranslator.com to calculate a target range of fat to consume, including limits on saturated fat, trans fats, and cholesterol. Try to limit your saturated fat intake to no more than one-third of the total fat you eat. That means that if you eat about 45 grams of total fat per day, try to eat less than 15 grams of saturated fat per day. Avoid trans fat completely. And if you have diabetes or a cardiovascular disease, you should consult a nutrition professional to specify your unique fat needs.

■ cholesterol Limit your cholesterol to 300 mg per day if you don't have high cholesterol levels, but keep under 200 mg if your LDL (bad cholesterol) is high or you are taking medication to lower your cholesterol. Your body makes approximately 1000 mg of cholesterol per day, so it's fine if you don't consume much cholesterol. Try limiting your beef intake to no more than one meal per week. A 3-ounce portion of trimmed lean sirloin steak and a 3-ounce cod filet both contain 47 mg of cholesterol, so watch your portions of protein from all animal sources to keep cholesterol consumption at your target level.

■ calcium   The reference Daily Value used for nutrition labeling is 1000 mg as a target for adults and children over the age of four years. These references are designed to meet the needs of most individuals, but after menopause women need an additional 200 mg or a total of 1200 mg to meet their needs. If you don't consume dairy products or soy products with added calcium, you may need a calcium supplement to get these recommended amounts daily. See the high-calcium food group in Appendix B for calcium content of a variety of foods and supplements.

■ vitamin D   This vitamin has been the center of attention in the nutrition world recently, and there is controversy about the amount a given individual needs. Since more individuals are being tested, I am seeing more clients who have low blood levels of this important vitamin. The reference Daily Value is currently 400 International Units (IU) per day, but some experts recommend 800 to 2,000 IU of vitamin D per day, especially during winter months for those individuals who live in northern climates or who are at risk of a deficiency. Check with your healthcare provider if you're not sure how much to take. Risk of vitamin D insufficiency increases as you age; for example, by the time you are seventy, your body is 75 percent less able to convert the vitamin D in your skin to the active form. And it's also nearly impossible to get enough of this sunshine vitamin from food, so taking a supplement might be necessary to top off the amount you get in your diet. And if your doctor tests you and finds that your blood level of vitamin D is low, he or she may want to prescribe a mega-dose for a short time to restore you to a healthy level. Also, being a smoker, taking certain medications, or drinking alcohol to excess can interfere with your absorption of vitamin D and indicate the need for supplementation.

■ iron   Intake of this mineral varies with age and gender. While men need only 6 mg per day, women need 8 mg prior to menopause but only 5 mg after menopause. Because your absorption of iron from plant-based foods can be reduced by other substances in food that you eat on the same day, the Daily Value for iron is 18. Pregnant women need the most iron (22 mg per day). The needs of lactating women return to the pre-pregnancy level. Since animal sources are the highest in iron and the iron they contain may be easier to absorb, those individuals following a vegetarian diet may need to pay more attention to plant foods rich in iron or take a multivitamin that contains 100 percent of the Daily Value.

■ vitamin C   Adult women and men need 60 mg vitamin C per day, but pregnant women need 70 mg and lactating women need 100 mg per day. Selecting fruits and vegetables that are good sources of vitamin C daily will help to meet this recommendation, but when calories are limited a supplement may be necessary. Most multivitamin supplements provide 60 mg in a daily dose. Avoid mega-doses unless you consult with your health care provider. Food sources of vitamin C are noted in the Food Groups list in Appendix B.

■ vitamin A   This vitamin should be included at least every other day. The Daily Value for vitamin A is 5,000 IU per day or 35,000 IU per week. Because your body can store this vitamin you don't need to consume it each day. You can eat fruits and vegetables that are very rich sources of vitamin A (such as sweet potatoes or carrots) three or four times per week and be sure you are getting enough. Good foods that are high in this vitamin are noted in the Food Groups list in Appendix B. If you do take a multivitamin, avoid those that contain more than 100 percent of the Daily Value.

Fluid Intake — Water is the most essential nutrient, but how do you know how much to drink each day? If you are eating appropriate amounts of fruits and vegetables (which contain up to 80 percent water) you may be getting about one-fifth of the fluids you need each day from produce. But if you are eating mostly dry foods such as snack foods, protein, and fats you may be getting very little water in the solid foods. Although you can count the fluids in coffee, tea, milk, and soups, you shouldn't count alcoholic beverages as part of your daily requirement. And your fluid intake should also be spaced out during the day. Women should consume 9 cups of fluid per day; men should consume 13 cups of fluid per day. Good food targets in Appendix A include recommended amounts of fluid based on the amount of food you consume.

If you are physically active you may need 1–3 cups of additional water or fluid each day, especially before, during, and after exercise. I recommend using filtered tap water rather than bottled water, since many bottled waters are simply bottled tap water. And the amount of raw materials and energy used to bottle this water leaves a big carbon footprint on the earth. Get yourself a good glass or stainless steel insulated cup to carry your water when you are away from home.

■ alcohol   Alcohol is not a required nutrient but it does contain calories. In fact it contains nearly twice the calories of sugar. It can be consumed as part of your choice calories. Women should not consume more than 1 serving per day and men should drink no more than 2 servings per day. Serving sizes vary depending on the drink, but in general 12 ounces of beer, 5 ounces of wine, or 1 ounce of distilled liquor would count as 1 serving. Keep in mind that many mixed drinks may contain 2 or more servings in a single glass, and juices, cream, or other ingredients will also contribute extra calories.

■ antioxidants   Current research suggests that foods high in antioxidants may help prevent many diseases, but the studies are far from conclusive on exactly what amounts of these substances found in food are necessary. In the meantime, a diet that includes a wide variety of vegetables, fruits, nuts, beans, and whole grains is going to provide a significant amount of antioxidants. The various pigments that color fruits and vegetables are indicative of the antioxidant type as well as content, so varying the colors on your plate may be more beneficial in keeping us healthy than taking supplements or limiting our choices to just a few foods that are promoted as high in antioxidants.

Meal and Snack Planning
Managing Time, Money, and Health

At my house the main discussion at lunch was what we were going to have for dinner.
—Paul Lynde (1926–1982)

PLANNING IS THE STARTING POINT for achieving any worthwhile goal or embarking on any journey. Having a route mapped out does not mean that you can't take a side trip if you find an unexpected point of interest to visit. But the map will help you get to your ultimate destination without getting lost along the way.

Not everyone's plan will be the same, and not everyone's destination will be the same. So the ideas presented here are designed to help you to evaluate how you eat now and to encourage you to think about what you want to eat and be ready to commit to a general plan for every day.

Planning your at-home meals, your snacks, and your away-from-home meals can be done on a daily or weekly basis, depending on how often you shop, on how well-stocked your kitchen is, and on your lifestyle. Begin by developing a repertoire of five to seven dinner meals that you can always depend on, especially when life gets hectic and you don't even have time to think or plan. Always in a rush? Then have restaurant or menu choices planned in advance for occasions when eating out or taking out is a necessity. Even unplanned, unpredictable meals will improve as your habits and food choices become more natural and intuitive. Small, simple changes can make a big difference.

When I first met my clients Natalie and David, they were eating out or getting take-out meals nearly every night. They have two children under the age of three, and both parents work full time. They wanted to lose weight and give their young children better eating habits, but it was obvious that cooking at home every night would be too drastic a change for them. As we talked about what

> Begin by developing a repertoire of five to seven dinner meals that you can always depend on, especially when life gets hectic and you don't even have time to think or plan.

changes would be realistic for them at the start, they agreed to have dinner at home two nights a week. Next we worked on selecting different items at their favorite restaurants and take-out places using menus and online nutrition information that these restaurants provide. After several months, they are now eating out only twice a week. They have both started losing weight, and they and their children are eating more fruit and vegetables, which they were rarely getting with their take-out dinners.

Redesigning Your Meals

ready TO BEGIN PLANNING?

I RECOMMEND SITTING DOWN WITH A BLANK SHEET OF PAPER or a blank calendar and actually writing down what you will have for dinner for a week. Or if you really don't feel creative, simply keep track of your usual lunch or dinner meals for a week or two. Don't change everything at once; for example, you could add a second vegetable to your usual dinner even if it's a frozen entrée. You can also go to www.3DYourWholeLife.com to view more sample menus or to print out a meal planning worksheet.

When planning dinner, consider starting with the entrée (usually lean protein or whole grain item) first, for example, chicken legs, black beans, eggs, fish, and so on. Make the protein approximately a quarter of the food on your plate. Then you can select vegetables that are compatible with the entrée, including items from each of the color groups each day whenever possible:

blue and purple   green (pale or dark green)
white   yellow and orange   red

Plan to have **at least half your plate full of vegetables.** You'll be increasing the visual appeal of your meal. And choosing some foods from each of the color groups insures not only a good variety of vitamins and minerals, but also each color of pigment provides a different cluster of antioxidants that are so important for optimal health. Each day's menu should include a good source of vitamin C (like citrus fruit or bell peppers) and at least 4 servings each week of a vegetable or fruit (carrots, butternut squash, spinach and other dark greens, cantaloupe, or mango) that is high in vitamin A. Try including a fruit in your main meals or snacks.

Planning Possibilities

Pick a day each week and set aside thirty minutes to plan what you will eat for the upcoming week. Consider your schedule and that of your dinner partners. Start with one meal a day, for instance, dinner. Write down your plan and keep it visible in the kitchen so that you can refer to it every day.

Have meal kits bundled together for quick last-minute meals. For example, take a look at the recipe for "Shrimp, Cannellini, and Tomatoes." Keep a copy of the recipe with some canned beans and tomatoes to avoid having to locate it when you're rushed. Keeping frozen cooked shrimp on hand completes the recipe. You might even consider storing the ingredients and a copy of the recipe in the dish or equipment you'll need to make it.

Take non-perishable snacks with you when traveling or if you have limited access to good choices when away from home, such as a snack bag of nuts and dried fruit. Have snacks pre-portioned to avoid eating a larger portion if you're very hungry or stressed. Planning the portion ahead makes it less likely that you'll overeat. If you don't eat the snack immediately, it will not spoil or expire that day.

Check online for menus and nutritional information from your favorite restaurants. If your local restaurant doesn't have a website, you might find that the national chains list typical menu items such as pizza, pasta, salads, and sandwiches on their websites. Use this information to analyze the kinds of meals you are ordering. Look for healthier options and plan to order something different next time you dine out.

Next to consider are the whole grains and starches that you will include. What texture and taste will complement the protein and produce you've planned? Include at least 3 servings of whole grain each day and make at least half your grains "whole." For example, if you usually eat 6 servings of starches such as bread or cereals, then make sure that at least 3 servings are from whole-grain sources. Of course, you can choose all whole grains to make your meals even healthier. Check the Food Group lists in Appendix B for serving sizes to evaluate the foods that you usually eat. For example, if you eat a cup of oatmeal every morning, you'll already be getting 2 servings of whole grain, since each ½ cup gets credit as 1 whole grain. The portions listed in the Food Groups lists in Appendix B are not necessarily the right portions for everyone, but they can help you evaluate the amounts of what you are eating and what you could include in your meal planning. Having a slice of tomato and 1 leaf of lettuce on your sandwich would not be enough to count as a serving of vegetable, although garnishes of fruits and vegetables could certainly add up over the course of an entire day to an additional serving.

Your dinner meal is only a part of your daily food intake. So you might want to jot down what you eat for two or three days (including the amount) just to see what you are consuming in a typical day. Be sure to include restaurant meals, school lunches, tasting food while cooking, snacks at meetings or while in the car, and any beverages or condiments, so that you will have a good snapshot. Next, using the good food targets in Appendix A, determine how your intake of the core foods compares with the recommended servings. Women should use the 1600-Calorie level guideline for comparison. Men should compare daily foods with the 2200-Calorie guideline for core foods. Feel free to use another calorie level for comparison if you have specific nutritional needs. For example, individuals with diabetes who are counting carbohydrates should consult with their diabetes educator or registered dietitian before changing their customary meal plan. And if you are very active physically or work out intensely, you'll need more good food than the average person who isn't seriously exercising.

On the next page is an example of how portions of the same menu might differ for a typical woman needing about 1600 Calories and a typical man needing approximately 2200.

Menu Comparison*

Breakfast	1600 Cal.	2200 Cal.
Oven-baked Oatmeal	1 serving	1 serving
Nonfat Milk	1 cup	1 cup
Pink Grapefruit Sections	½ cup	½ cup
Lunch		
Thin Crust Pizza	1 slice	2 slices
Green Grapes	15 (3 ounces)	15 (3 ounces)
Broccoli Slaw (oil and lemon)	2 cups	2 cups
Afternoon Snack		
Strawberry Greek Yogurt	6 ounces	6 ounces
Tangelo	1	1
Dinner		
Classic Roasted Chicken	3 ounces	4 ounces
Whole Berry Cranberry Sauce	2 tablespoons	2 tablespoons
Roasted Roots	1 serving	2 servings
Fresh Asparagus	1 cup	1-1/2 cups
Whole Wheat Roll	------	1
Fruit Crisp	1 serving	1 serving
Evening Snack		
Air Popped Popcorn	3 cups	6 cups

* Foods that appear in bold are available in the recipe section of Chapter 1

Below is the nutrient content of each menu. Notice that not only is the calorie count different but other nutrients such as fat, fiber and sodium are proportionately higher in the 2200-Calorie menu portions. And although the nutrition facts label does not separate the amount of added sugars from the total sugar content, there are actually only 26 total grams of added sugar (from the yogurt, the fruit crisp, and 1 gram in the pizza crust). That's far less than the 36 grams or less per day that I mentioned earlier. The remainder of the sugar is natural sugar from whole unprocessed foods such as milk, fruit, vegetables, and whole grains. These are some of the very foods that contribute to the excellent fiber content of this menu.

1600-Calorie Menu

Nutrition Facts

Serving Size (1793g)
Servings Per Container

Amount Per Serving

Calories 1610   Calories from Fat 480

	% Daily Value*
Total Fat 54g	83%
Saturated Fat 19g	95%
Trans Fat 0g	
Cholesterol 130mg	43%
Sodium 910mg	38%
Total Carbohydrate 223g	74%
Dietary Fiber 30g	120%
Sugars 116g	
Protein 78g	

Vitamin A 290%	•	Vitamin C 470%
Calcium 120%	•	Iron 60%

*Percent Daily Values are based on a 2,000 calorie diet. Your daily values may be higher or lower depending on your calorie needs:

		Calories:	2,000	2,500
Total Fat	Less than		65g	80g
Saturated Fat	Less than		20g	25g
Cholesterol	Less than		300mg	300mg
Sodium	Less than		2,400mg	2,400mg
Total Carbohydrate			300g	375g
Dietary Fiber			25g	30g

Calories per gram:
Fat 9 • Carbohydrate 4 • Protein 4

2200-Calorie Menu

Nutrition Facts

Serving Size (2273g)
Servings Per Container

Amount Per Serving

Calories 2220   Calories from Fat 670

	% Daily Value*
Total Fat 75g	115%
Saturated Fat 24g	120%
Trans Fat 0g	
Cholesterol 160mg	53%
Sodium 1580mg	66%
Total Carbohydrate 307g	102%
Dietary Fiber 44g	176%
Sugars 130g	
Protein 107g	

Vitamin A 480%	•	Vitamin C 530%
Calcium 140%	•	Iron 90%

*Percent Daily Values are based on a 2,000 calorie diet. Your daily values may be higher or lower depending on your calorie needs:

		Calories:	2,000	2,500
Total Fat	Less than		65g	80g
Saturated Fat	Less than		20g	25g
Cholesterol	Less than		300mg	300mg
Sodium	Less than		2,400mg	2,400mg
Total Carbohydrate			300g	375g
Dietary Fiber			25g	30g

Calories per gram:
Fat 9 • Carbohydrate 4 • Protein 4

Remember, you don't have to count calories to plan healthy meals, but **you will need to count servings** of the core foods until you get the hang of it.

If your usual meals and snacks don't add up to the total recommended servings of the core foods, make a note of which foods you want to include more often. A client of mine, Nancy, thought she was eating a good diet and healthy foods. When she kept a food log for a week, she discovered that she was eating excessive amounts of fruit but not eating many vegetables. To get back in balance, Nancy started to substitute raw vegetables in place of fruit at lunch. And she began by buying a platter of assorted raw vegetables at the supermarket each week and placing it on a shelf at eye level in her refrigerator. **Simple changes** like the one Nancy made can lead to big improvements in your eating habits.

The lower-calorie menu comes up a bit short on iron, providing only 60 percent of the Daily Value. Since women generally need less food (and foods contain iron) than men and they need more iron before they reach menopause, it's more difficult to meet their iron needs without taking a multivitamin or overeating red meat. Choosing foods that are enriched with iron or foods that are naturally high in iron, such as dark green leafy vegetables, dried plums, dark meat chicken, and shellfish is also a great option.

Use the three-color rule

Aim for at least three different colors on your plate for main meals. This is an easy way to get a variety of nutrients and flavors into each meal you serve, and it provides eye appeal as well. Vegetables and fruits can provide color and improve a beige or white meal nutritionally. Expand beyond pasta, potatoes, chicken, rice, and cheese!

Meal Planning Quiz

- Do you know at 5 PM what you will be having for dinner?
- Could you assemble a well-balanced meal if you were home in a storm and couldn't get to the market?
- Do you make your lunch for the next day at dinner?

If you've answered yes to all of the above— congratulations!

You are a mindful eater and a good planner!

- Do you run out the door in the morning without enough time to eat something?
- Do you have vegetables only at dinner and fruits only at breakfast?
- Is cooking food the last thing you want to think about as you're driving home at night?

If you've answered yes to any of these questions,

you need to spend a few minutes each day on planning
to avoid impulsive eating or
neglecting to include all the healthy foods that your body needs...

Choosing Recipes
Old Favorites and New Ideas

Food is so primal, so essential a part of our lives, often the mere sharing of recipes with strangers turns them into good friends.
—Jasmine Heller

MY MISSION AS A REGISTERED DIETITIAN AND NUTRITIONIST is to inform and inspire my clients to eat in healthier ways, so I'm always looking for ideas for new recipes or better versions of old favorites. I own hundreds of recipe books and even more volumes on food and food customs. I have subscriptions to many popular food magazines as well as to online recipe websites. I find recipes in the food pages of newspapers and receive favorite recipes from friends and clients. I've even found them in novels and gardening books. But I am also discerning in looking for well-formulated recipes that are packed with healthy ingredients, and for every recipe I evaluate and save, I reject a hundred others. Other vital criteria such as the impact on the planet God has given us, how and where the ingredients are grown, and the general ethics of consuming enough food to nourish us and our families without eating more than we need, enter into my decisions about ingredients, recipes, and portions. These should also be factors you consider when making decisions about what you eat.

In addition to providing tasty and nutritious recipes for my clients, I am motivated to find delicious recipes for myself. I like to combine healthy foods with savory herbs and spices to achieve the most flavor and the most nutrition I can from the foods available. I love nothing better than to spend a Saturday shopping for great food, preparing it well, and sharing it with family and friends at the end of the day.

Yet with my busy schedule during the week, when I spend long hours helping my clients and patients in the office, I need to have meals planned in advance and ready to assemble quickly at the end of the day. As much as I love to cook, sometimes my husband will do the cooking or we'll share the cooking depending on a given day's schedule. As the youngest in his family and the only son, he did not learn to cook beyond the most basic skills, but now with practice not only can he put a wonderful meal on the table, but also he can read a recipe and know if it will work well for us while being healthy and tasty. This chapter is about just that: making decisions about which recipes you choose and prepare. And to begin, a good recipe meets the following basic criteria:

1. It matches the skill level of the cook.
2. It satisfies the person who prepares it as well as those consuming the dish.
3. It contributes to the goal of eating right.
4. It's cost effective —it meets the budget of the cook or the family.
5. It can be prepared in the time available.

How to Evaluate a Recipe: Questions to Ask

What are the 3 ingredients that are present in the largest quantities?

Usually recipes present the ingredient list in the order in which you will use the ingredients during preparation. This is quite different from looking at the ingredient list on a food label, which lists the ingredients by quantity. You can still use the recipe's ingredient list to evaluate its nutrient content by looking at the 3 ingredients that are present in the greatest quantities. For instance, if you are evaluating a vegetable soup recipe, you would add up the total amount of vegetables required to make the stated number of portions. Soup recipes are often written for 6–12 servings per recipe. So if the recipe calls for 2 carrots, 2 stalks of celery, and 3 cups of cabbage in a recipe that makes 12 cups, there are not enough raw vegetables to count as a serving, if a serving is 1 cup. Here's a tip for increasing the health factor of a recipe: If the soup calls for sautéing onions in butter, you can easily substitute olive oil, and chances are that you could use half the amount of fat and not notice the difference in flavor.

What is the cooking method?

Is the food baked, broiled, roasted, fried, steamed, grilled, microwaved, poached, or sautéed? Does it cook all day in a slow cooker? Does it need to be marinated ahead of time? The cooking method can add calories in the form of fat, or it may actually encourage the dripping of fat from the food, such as broiled meat or fish. Moist cooking such as poaching or braising will make tough foods such as inexpensive lean cuts of meat more tender than roasting or baking them (see the Five Spice Pork Pot Roast recipe).

What is the preparation and cooking time?

Can you prepare the ingredients ahead of time or pre-cook part of the recipe to save time before dinner (see Roasted Summer Vegetables recipe) or breakfast (see Oven-baked Oatmeal recipe)? Peeling and chopping vegetables in advance can make assembling a stir-fry at the end of the day a real breeze. You can even mix the condiments or cooking sauce the night before or in the morning and have it ready in the refrigerator to add to the stir-fry. The actual cooking time may be less than 15 minutes once the ingredients are ready. You can cook the rice in the microwave to save time or you can cook it in large batches and freeze portions to quickly reheat when you need it. Cooking ahead in large batches can also save energy and cut down on your utility bill. Microwaving to reheat food prepared ahead uses only a minimum of energy. And since it's difficult to find convenience entrées that contain whole grain or do not contain high amounts of sodium, making a recipe ahead and freezing it can be a simple way to eat good food even on your busiest days.

Is the nutrient content included in the recipe?

Many recipe books, magazines, and websites routinely include some basic nutrient content along with the yield (servings) of the recipe. Some also include the servings from the various food groups or diabetic exchanges. You can simply estimate the numbers of servings of meat, vegetables, or fat by dividing the main ingredients by the number of servings. For instance, if the recipe calls for 4 6-ounce portions of boneless skinless chicken breast to serve 4 portions, you will be cooking a total of 24 ounces of chicken. If you want to eat a 3-ounce portion of chicken, then you only need to eat a half portion. If the recipe uses 2 tablespoons of olive oil, then your 3-ounce portion will probably also provide less than 1 teaspoon of fat. If the nutrient content is provided in the recipe, remember to evaluate the portion you will actually consume. If a recipe calls for a 4-ounce apple per person and you will be using 8-ounce apples, then the nutrient content will be proportionately higher—or your serving could be half of the large apple.

If the nutrient content is not listed in the recipe and you would like to know the actual calories, you can use one of the online resources listed in the Resources section. Or you may have a food composition book or calorie-counting book that lists the nutrients contained in the main ingredients. You can also refer to the Food Groups information in Appendix B.

Can you lighten the recipe without changing the characteristics of the finished product?

Perhaps you could substitute low-fat cheese for full-fat cheese. Maybe you could sauté the vegetables in half the oil specified or use a few tablespoons of broth instead. You could substitute nonfat plain Greek yogurt for sour cream. Or you might omit or reduce the salt in a soup or entrée to lower the sodium content. Be careful substituting ingredients in baked goods; the chemistry is often a delicate balance and is not as forgiving as a soup if you make changes in the ingredients.

What is the skill level necessary to make the recipe?

The cook's skill level is an important consideration in recipe selection. A simple elegant dish does not always require sophisticated skills. Some recipes are categorized or rated by skill level but most are not, although a recipe that indicates the time it takes to prepare it can be a clue to the complexity of the dish. Some recipes assume basic cooking skills or the mastery of particular techniques, but they may not specifically be stated in the instructions.

Just like reading the roadmap or programming your GPS before starting a trip, you should read the recipe thoroughly before you even include it in your dinner plans for tonight. Here are some other important questions to ask yourself before deciding to make a dish:

- Do you have the ingredients on hand or will you need to buy more to make it?
- Do you have the equipment and/or appliances to achieve the right outcome?
- How long will it take you to prepare it?
- Can the recipe be partially or totally prepared in advance?
- Will leftovers be able to be frozen or will they need to be consumed quickly?
- Will the recipe be served on its own, such as a slow-cooker entrée? Or will it be part of a more complicated menu?
- Is there a way to improve the recipe's health benefits, such as doubling the amount of vegetables in a casserole or soup?
- Do you need to adjust the serving size?
- Can you garnish the dish with fruit or vegetables to add color, appeal, texture, or nutritional value? Even a tablespoon of chopped parsley, basil, or cilantro will add vitamins, minerals, and antioxidants. And it will enhance the appearance of the humblest entrée and add to the complexity of the flavor. A small slice of melon on the plate with a sandwich can be visually appealing—it can be counted as half a serving of fruit and amounts to only a few calories. A fruit or vegetable garnish also can serve to cover the plate where in the past you may have chosen chips or French fries, and it can also provide the crunch you may be used to having.

If the recipe is time-consuming, can you add a quick side dish to reduce your work? If you are making a labor-intensive entrée, try using 2 frozen vegetables for quick and colorful sides. Or buy a butternut squash that's already peeled and chopped, which will cook quickly without requiring your constant attention. It's simpler and less stressful to devote yourself to one great dish than to try to orchestrate a complicated meal, unless you are an experienced cook.

Try new creations: Once a week take out items from the refrigerator, freezer, or cabinets that you want to use and create a soup or casserole or something totally new. Use search engines on the Web to find uses for those foods. For example, a search for a recipe on www.epicurious.com for recipes containing celery, mushrooms, and chicken produces a long list starting with chicken stew, various chicken soups, and interesting entrées.

Even though I have hundreds of recipe books, sometimes this method is quicker and can trigger ideas that are outside my usual repertoire of cooking. See, you don't have to revert to your recipe using that canned "Cream of . . . " soup, which is not going to contribute much to the dish in the way of nutrients except excess sodium and empty calories.

Tips for Making the Most of Recipes

- Pick recipes that include a vegetable, fruit, lean protein, healthy fat, or a whole grain as 1 of the 3 main ingredients.
- Make note of recipes that you would like to repeat in the future. Keep a file of clippings or recipe cards, or archive online recipes for future use. There are many recipe websites that include a personalized "recipe box" feature. Or you can optically scan recipe clippings and store them on your computer.
- If you choose a complex dish as part of a meal, keep the other items simple—an elaborate vegetable dish can be paired with quickly broiled meat, poultry, or fish. If you're making a complex curry, then choose plain rice and a fresh fruit to accompany it.
- Evaluate the portion size listed in a recipe. Is it the amount that you, your family, and friends will eat? Will you need to make more or less?
- Consider doubling recipes that will freeze well for another meal, or plan to use extra for a lunch or snack the next day.

PREPARING

Getting Your Kitchen in Order

First comes thought; then organization of that thought, into ideas and plans; then transformation of those plans into reality. The beginning, as you will observe, is in your imagination.

—Napoleon Hill (1883–1970)

ORGANIZATION IS CRITICAL for planning and preparing healthy meals, but we each need to find a system that works for us. For example, I have a friend who stores all of her kitchen spices and ingredients alphabetically, so that she is able to find them immediately. On the other end of the spectrum I discovered that another friend stores her supplies in utter chaos behind the closed cupboards of her gourmet kitchen, claiming she knows exactly where everything is. Most of us are probably somewhere in between, and there's no one "right way" to organize a kitchen, even as there's no perfect kitchen layout for every cook and every household.

An organized kitchen is not a matter of having the designer kitchen cabinets, the latest refrigerator, or the most attractive storage containers. It's really about managing *your* kitchen, *your* budget, *your* time, *your* ingredients, and *your* equipment in order to produce healthy and delicious meals and quick wholesome snacks when they are needed. Sometimes that may mean simplifying your kitchen and clearing away items that you seldom need or use only on special occasions. And sometimes it may mean purchasing some additional equipment that will help you in the production of good food. In any case, having an organized space in which to prepare your meals and snacks will not only insure that you will eat more nutritionally but also enjoy the peace and calmness of spirit that it will bring you. Having an organized kitchen can help you cultivate the grace to receive divine inspiration for your meals.

> There's no one "right way" to organize a kitchen, even as there's no perfect kitchen layout for every cook and every household.

Just as Robert Browning's poem says, "God's in his heaven—All's right with the world," I find that when my kitchen is in good order the whole house seems to function on a higher level.

I recently added a small freezer in the garage to store extra food that I want to save for future meals and to take advantage of sales on my favorite perishable items. I found this energy-efficient freezer on sale and researched the energy use, which amounts to an additional $30 per year, a small carbon footprint. This additional stored food also helps to cut down on unnecessary trips to the grocery store; since I live in a semi-rural area, given the high price of gasoline, the freezer will probably pay for itself over the next year.

That isn't to say that bulk food purchases are always the best approach. Buying larger packages may seem like a bargain, but it also may mean you are likely to eat more than you need. So if you buy at a food warehouse or discount store, buy only as much as you need, or be sure to freeze or store the extras as soon as you unpack the groceries.

> If you buy at a food warehouse or discount store, buy only as much as you need, or be sure to freeze or store the extras as soon as you unpack the groceries.

When we think about what we'd like in a well-organized kitchen, some of us are overwhelmed by having too much food on hand. Others are stressed about not having enough of the right ingredients available at the end of a long day. If your organizational style is the latter, consider using a closet or shelves that can accommodate staple items and foods that are only occasionally needed. Organization is simpler when extra items don't clutter your daily workspace and kitchen cabinets and counters.

Now let's take a long look at your kitchen, your habits, and your cooking environment—as well as your equipment.

Kitchen Q&A

Are the refrigerator and freezer clean and well organized?

I recommend a thorough cleaning of your refrigerator every month. That means taking out everything and washing the shelves, doors, and gaskets (the rubber edging around the doors). Keeping up with spills as they happen will make major cleaning much easier.

Your freezer should be organized at least once a month, or before a big shopping trip. Freezer burn may mean that you haven't properly packaged the food, or it may have spent too much time in the freezer. Items such as meats that are showing freezer burn should be used as soon as possible in dishes such as soups, stews, or casseroles. The burn doesn't mean they're spoiled but that they will be dry and will benefit from moist, low, slow heat.

Do you utilize the "first in, first out" principle to rotate foods?

When you're in a hurry, you may be tempted to place an item in the first available space in the freezer or refrigerator. Take an extra minute to pull the package of frozen peas that is already in the freezer to the front and place the newest package behind it.

Do you label and date foods after opening packages?

Keep some labels or masking tape and a waterproof marker handy in the kitchen. Get into the habit of marking leftovers and opened packages of staple items. It's so easy to forget what's in that bag in the bottom of the freezer and when you put it there. Labeling and dating will help you avoid wasting precious food items.

Are there any foods that are beyond their expiration date? Are there any food items that should be used in the next 24 hours or frozen for future use? Are there any foods that should be discarded?

Check your refrigerator every day to see if any food items are getting close to their expiration or "best used by" date. Incorporate them into today's meals or snacks to avoid wasting them. Before you complete your grocery list, I also recommend checking your dry storage area to see if any items should be used that week. Discard any items that have expired or are suspect (never consume food from a can that is bulging or leaking). Check your freezer weekly also.

Are potentially hazardous foods such as raw meats or fish stored in a way that prevents contamination of other foods with bacteria?

Always store raw meats on the bottom shelf of the refrigerator. Place them on a tray or in a bowl or plastic bag to prevent the meat juices from spilling and contaminating raw foods.

Is there a thermometer inside your refrigerator, freezer, and storage closet or cupboards to check the temperature?

Built-in thermometers may not always be accurate, so place a small hanging thermometer in the refrigerator (target temperature is less than 40 degrees Fahrenheit) and the freezer (target temperature is less than 0 degrees Fahrenheit). Check it each day to make sure your food is being stored in a safe range. Food in dry storage is best kept at 50–70 degrees.

Are all packages of pantry staples airtight and impervious to insects and pests?

I recommend airtight plastic, ceramic, or glass containers rather than plastic bags for storing grains, cereals, pasta, or chocolate. Pantry moths can eat through a plastic bag and contaminate your grains; rodents will eat through a flimsy package to get to chocolate (and just about everything else). So avoid having to discard expensive food by packaging it securely each time you store it.

Do you keep your recipe sources in the kitchen or readily available?

Which sources do you routinely use? Pick three to five favorite cookbooks or magazines to keep handy in the kitchen or at your desk or near your computer. Make copies of favorite recipes to store with key ingredients to prepare quick last-minute dishes with a minimum of stress and time.

Essential Equipment

Simplify and organize the cooking equipment you use. Keep frequently used utensils and equipment handy to the cooking area. Remove seldom used items and store in an area that is accessible when they are needed (closets, on storage shelves, in the basement or garage).

Your need for equipment will depend on factors such as your cooking skill and the number of people in the household. Large households will require larger saucepans and cutting boards. Singles and couples will cook more efficiently with smaller capacity pots and pans.

A Baker's Dozen of Equipment Necessary to Prepare a Variety of Good Food

1. Knives: 1 each paring, boning, serrated slicer, large wedge knife, and a sharpener
2. Standing type shredder or a mandolin slicer/shredder and a rasp for grating nutmeg or lemons
3. Saucepans in a variety of sizes from 1 quart to 1 gallon
4. Heavy covered casserole or Dutch oven
5. 1–2 gallon stockpot (can be used to cook pasta and soups)
6. Cutting boards that are dishwasher safe (easy to sanitize)
7. Heat-tolerant flexible spatulas
8. Heavyweight roasting pan
9. Heavyweight rimmed cookie sheets or half-size sheet pans
10. Durable salad spinner
11. Sharp vegetable peelers, 1 narrow and 1 wide
12. Thermometers for refrigerator, freezer, dry storage, and oven
13. Instant-read thermometer to check temperatures of meats, reheated leftovers, and other critical cooking and serving temperatures

Extra tip: A versatile piece of kitchen equipment is the black cast iron pan, the original non-stick skillet. The pans can be used on the stove or in the oven. I have them in several sizes (6 to 14 inches in diameter). They retain heat and seal in flavors without much added fat. Never use detergent on a cast iron pan—it will pick up the taste of soap. Clean the skillet while it's still warm with coarse kosher salt and a cloth, rinse, and then wipe completely dry before storing.

Recommended Utensils and Portion Guides

- Set of dry-ingredient measuring cups that include ⅛, ¼, ⅓, ½, ⅔, ¾, and 1 cup measures
- Set of metal measuring spoons that include ⅛, ¼, ½, and 1 teaspoon, and ½ and 1 tablespoon, if possible
- Pyrex® glass measuring cups for liquid measurements—1 cup, 2 cup, 1 quart, and 2 quart sizes. The 2-quart size can double as a measuring bowl.
- Ice cream scoops in sizes from 1 ounce to 4 ounces
- Ladles in sizes—1 ounce, 2 ounces, 4 ounces, and 8 ounces
- 1–2 ounce shot glass for measuring nuts and small amounts of liquids
- Food scale (preferably digital)

Appliances

During the course of my personal and professional life as a cook, I have prepared food in a range of cooking environments. From the coal-fired cast iron stove of my grandparents' kitchen to a campfire in the mountains, from the small kitchen of my first apartment to my current kitchen that I designed, from my office mini-kitchen to commercial kitchens of my clients, I have always managed to utilize the appliances available to produce nutritious and enjoyable meals.

In my practice as a nutritionist, I see individuals who have only a microwave and a hotplate as well as those who have well-equipped gourmet kitchens. There is no excuse not to eat right in any cooking environment if you plan accordingly. Having every latest appliance does not guarantee eating well or living well. Beyond having some means of refrigeration and a stovetop form of cooking, the other choices are up to you, depending on your style of cooking, your budget, and your expertise. For example, I have been baking bread for years but I don't use a bread machine; I knead the dough by hand, let it rise in a warm spot in the kitchen, and bake it in the oven. I find that being in close touch with the bread dough I am preparing is one of the fringe benefits of cooking from scratch. Good food is not only physically nourishing but also spiritually satisfying as well. In other words, don't let the equipment do all the work.

Some of the appliances that you will find useful to prepare the recipes in this book and from other sources are:

- Microwave oven
- Toaster or toaster oven
- Broiler
- Outdoor grill or a stovetop grill
- Food processor, 1 medium to large capacity and 1 mini-size (optional)
- Handheld or standing mixer
- Handheld immersion blender and/or full-size blender
- Spice grinder (or coffee grinder used only for spices)
- Full-size slow cooker (6–8 quart) or mini-Crock-Pot (optional)
- Pressure cooker (optional)
- Countertop grill or panini press (optional)

Tableware: Plate and Bowl Sizes

Do you have dishware or china available in a variety of sizes? If you are trying to decrease your portions, it can be helpful to "downsize" the plates, bowls, and cups that you use for your meals. An oversized 10–12 inch dinner plate is going to look emptier than a 9-inch plate when you decrease your portions. Your current portions might be determined more by the size of the dish than by a conscious decision. And don't forget to look at the size of the bowls and glasses you're using every day. Can you downsize them as well?

Make sure your dinnerware is safe to use in the microwave if you are in the habit of heating plates of food in it—dishes that contain metallic trim or those with deep color pigments may not be safe to use in the microwave. Throw out any dish or glass that has cracks or chips since bacteria can grow more easily in them, and these damaged pieces can shatter in the microwave. I also recommend against using plastic in the microwave. Try

> If you are trying to decrease your portions it can be helpful to "downsize" the plates, bowls, and cups that you use for your meals.

to use only glass, ceramic, china, or other non-reactive containers to heat up foods. Remove all items from plastic bags or restaurant take-out containers before microwaving.

Look at your flatware as well. Consider the size of your flatware to see if you can downsize your fork or spoon. Sure, a soupspoon will hold more of the liquid than a teaspoon, but a smaller spoon may help you slow the pace of your eating. You might want to try using a demitasse spoon for dessert instead of a teaspoon. And chopsticks can be fun and provide another way to be slower and more deliberate as you eat your meal.

Tips for Keeping Your Kitchen Clean and Organized

- **daily** — Check the refrigerator for the freshness of produce and other perishables; keep a running list of items you will need on shopping day or sooner.
- **weekly** — Before grocery shopping, take inventory of refrigerator and freezer contents, discard items that have expired or spoiled, empty fruit and vegetable drawers and wash out before replacing with usable items, and reorganize where items are stored. You may want to group items together that you tend to use at the same time. Don't forget to rotate the old items forward and place the newly purchased items in the back of the cabinet or shelf.
- **monthly** — Clean refrigerator and freezer. If you wipe up spills daily, you will not have to do a total cleaning as often. Clean and organize your dry storage on a regular basis. This will prevent items being forgotten on the back of the shelves.
- **seasonally** — Organize and clean exterior of spice and herb containers. Alphabetize to help in making a quick selection, or group items together that you use in the same recipes—for example, all the herbs used to make your Italian favorites or all the spices for curry together. Discard any items that are more than a year old, have lost their flavor or aroma, or look "off" in any way.
- **donate unneeded food** and equipment items to the local food pantry, your church, or a homeless shelter in your community.

Purchasing Good Food

Shipping is a terrible thing to do to vegetables.
They probably get jet-lagged, just like people.
—Elizabeth Barry

P LANNING MEETS PREPARATION AT THE GROCERY STORE. So try not to forget that shopping list you've written in advance or your coupons if you use them. And do as much research as you can at home before you get to the store. Examine the supermarket flyers or websites that feature the specials for the week as you plan your menu and your shopping list. Check your refrigerator and freezer to see if you need to add items to your list of staples or if you need to use something that you already have on hand. Try to develop a shopping strategy that works for you, your family, your time, and your budget. Use the following questions to help you get a plan in place.

How Often to Shop

I recommend shopping every week or two for staple items that you use regularly and more often for perishable items such as dairy products and produce. I find that my clients who shop on a scheduled day are most likely to have healthy food choices available during the week. It's probably because the routine of shopping on a particular day can insure that it will work with your weekly schedule, and you won't put it off until the cupboard is bare. Individuals who tell me that they shop when they "run out of things" run the risk of not having the right ingredients available, and they find themselves and their families skipping fruit and vegetables and resorting to refined foods when they run out of fresh foods.

Maybe it's just because nutrition is my profession and I love to cook that I enjoy going grocery shopping. If I had the time I would literally shop each day for that night's dinner. When I was staying with friends in the Netherlands, we would go to the market and purchase food for just a day or two. I would see people buying just enough to strap on the back of their bicycles for the ride home, and not too much to store in their small refrigerators. Whenever I have been in Italy, as well, I have seen the local women biking or walking to the market carrying shopping bags or pulling a small cart. While I was staying on the Isle of Capri, each morning when I went out for a walk I would see the same elderly women walking daily down the mountain into town with their baskets. On their return they would be laden with fresh fish, meat, bread, and lots of locally grown fruit and vegetables—walking briskly back up the mountain, never stopping. At the same time I would see tourists stopping to rest along the side of the steep roads as these elderly women energetically passed them. I'm sure that these women burned several hundred Calories by the time they got home and started to prepare their meals for the day!

In reality, though, most of us are lucky to get to the market once or twice a week, and we may have to drive to get there.

Where to Shop

My family and I will never take our supermarket for granted again after we traveled in the newly formed Republic of Hungary in 1990 and walked into a grocery store in a small town outside Budapest. My daughter was twelve at the time, and we all went in to see what sorts of products were on the shelves. To our surprise the store was lit only by two bare light bulbs hanging from the ceiling, the sparse cans of food were dusty, and the meat case held nothing but a few pieces of gray-looking meat. There was no fresh produce, because most people had gardens and grew their own vegetables. What a shift in our worldview as we headed back to our hotel!

There are many more sources of food available to us than ever before. Find the options that work best for you. Most Americans shop in supermarkets that carry about 30,000 different items. These "super stores" can be one-stop destinations for food, household supplies, prescriptions, and even plants and flowers. Discount bulk supermarket warehouses and shopping clubs have become more popular in the past ten years. They may carry fewer varieties of brands and often only items in large size or bulk packaging, which can offer better prices for those with a large household. I find that for some of my clients, buying larger portions than they can reasonably use at a meal or two can lead to overeating. Be aware of this risk if that is an issue for you.

Smaller markets such as convenience stores, greengrocers, fish markets, or butcher shops can be more expensive but can save time if you can get in, shop, and get out quickly. I prefer to shop for my fruits and vegetables at a local produce store. I like to be able to buy a single parsnip for soup or an orange beet for a salad. And I can buy just as much spinach or arugula as I need for dinner. The local or regional produce is not always as picture perfect as what the supermarket carries, but it generally doesn't disappoint in the flavor department. In summer I also shop the local farmers' markets for seasonal produce and homegrown and homemade items. And occasionally I will visit a specialty or gourmet food shop for special oils, vinegars, or teas that I can't find in my local supermarket.

Mail order and online shopping venues also give you the convenience and options of foods that you might not find in local stores. I sometimes order hard-to-find special ingredients for ethnic dishes online. And I like to give myself a "to me, from me" present now and then by ordering fruit such as pears or grapefruit directly from the growers. In many areas you can also order food from some supermarkets using online shopping and home delivery. You may not get to squeeze the avocados or smell the cantaloupe before you buy, but the time you save may be worth the delivery charge and the occasional less-than-perfect produce pick.

The very best source of produce may be right outside your back door. You may already be growing some herbs and vegetables yourself. I am lucky enough to have a vegetable garden that produces tomatoes, rhubarb, squash, and other bounty from God's green earth, but I also have an herb garden that provides me with at least eight months' of fresh seasonings and saves me lots of money. And I find that sharing my crops with others is an act of charity that is never refused. I can't beat the flavor when I walk out the back door and snip something fresh to enhance or garnish a meal. And if you don't have room to plant in the ground, try growing in containers like Earth Boxes (www.EarthBox.com), which resemble large window boxes. You can grow an incredible amount of produce using a simple potting mixture—no green thumb required. You may also have the option of growing a small plot in a community garden in your town. Or you may want to buy a share in a local farm, co-op, or greenhouse grower. Check out the increasing number of options that you have in your area.

If you shop in a traditional grocery store or supermarket, try to do most of your food buying around the perimeter of the store. Most stores are designed to locate the produce section at the entrance, then the fish, poultry, and meat at the back of the store, and the dairy and bakery in the last aisle to complete the "U" layout. The middle of the store in general contains more of the processed foods. Some exceptions are the whole-grain cereals, breads, crackers, and grains, frozen vegetables, spices, and various canned products. I like to buy a treat each weekend when I shop, so I go to the florist section first and put a lovely bunch of flowers or a plant in the seat of the shopping cart. Then I go to the produce section and start to select my fresh items. By the time I get to the fish and poultry section, I have a pretty colorful cartful of food.

If you shop in a traditional grocery store or supermarket, try to do most of your food buying around the perimeter of the store.

Send a Food Gift

I love to send fresh pears at Christmas to friends and family who live in other states. And I always send myself a box of pears too. There are many good sources of fruits, nuts, and other fresh foods that you may not find in your local grocery store. They may cost more but the quality of those pears is so wonderful that I find my family is much more excited about eating them. I also buy a case of grapefruit or oranges from the local high school students who sell them for fund-raising projects during the winter. They are shipped directly from Florida at the peak of the citrus season. Look for these opportunities in your community and your church.

Set your goal to purchase between 50 and 75 percent of your groceries from the perimeter of the store. And when you do push your cart up and down the aisles, take the time to read the labels on processed foods. If you buy canned vegetables, look for unsalted versions whenever possible (to keep your sodium intake at a reasonable level) and for canned fruits that don't have added sugars.

When choosing frozen vegetables, you'll save money and calories by selecting the items without added sauces or seasonings. Look at the ingredients list as well as the nutrition facts panel on the label. And beware the claims on foods that advertise themselves as health foods. For example, even if a cereal has a Whole Grain Stamp on the front of the box (indicating it supplies at least 8 grams of whole grain per serving), it still may be packed with extra sugar.

download more Good Food
information online at
www.3DYourWholeLife.com

How to Read a Food Label

- Check similar items' food labels to compare the nutritional content of similar foods. Look for items with the least added sugars, salt, and saturated fat.

- If an item different from what you usually buy is on sale, check the nutrition facts panel on the label to see if it is similar to what you usually buy. This will give you more flexibility than buying the same brand each time. Some store brands are identical to brand name products, but some have more sugar or are significantly different in other nutrients.

- Look at the ingredient list on processed or packaged food to see which 3 ingredients are present in the largest quantity: in general, these are where the majority of calories and other major nutrients come from. Be aware that sugar may also appear in several forms on labels such as high fructose corn syrup, dextrose, agave syrup, and brown rice syrup. These sugars may appear at first glance to be present in low amounts. By dividing them, the manufacturers move these items further down the list of ingredients. Also, be aware that "multigrain" doesn't mean "whole grain"; even if 15-grain bread sounds healthy, it may be made with a combination of 15 refined grains or 2–3 whole grains with a minuscule percentage of other grains.

- Read the nutrition description on the front of the package, too. Perhaps you'll see the word *light*. A food that has 50 percent less fat than the company's regular version or that has one-third fewer calories can be labeled *light*. But you'll want to keep in mind the simple nutrition principles you learned earlier to put this into perspective for your whole life. A light version of a high-fat premium ice cream may still be far higher in fat and calories than the regular, less expensive version of a store brand of ice cream—so compare side-by-side the nutrition facts labels on the packages and make your decision. Buyers beware!

■ Read the **health claim** on the front of the package. Although it may list the potential health benefits of one or more of the nutrients or the food itself, the manufacturer may be neglecting to tell you some other facts that may be important to you. For example, if a food is made with some whole grain or a healthy fat such as olive oil, that doesn't mean it isn't high in calories or highly processed. And remember that the manufacturer making the claim doesn't know what medications you take or how high your blood sugar or cholesterol is.

■ Avoid buying foods that contain **unhealthy ingredients:** monosodium glutamate (MSG), artificial food dyes, added sugars or corn syrup, artificial sweeteners, and trans fats.

■ Read the **nutrition facts panel** on the back or the side of the package. I recommend using these facts to comparison shop for items. In the example below you can see a regular mayonnaise and the light version produced by the same manufacturer. When comparing the two products side by side, you should look to see if the portions or serving sizes used for the label are the same. And then read down from the calories all the way to the percentage of vitamins and minerals listed below the bold black line. In this case the light product has only half the calories of the full-fat traditional version, even though the serving size is 2 grams larger. The fat content of the regular mayonnaise contains nearly the full amount of added fat recommended for an entire day for the average woman and two-thirds of the recommended fat intake for the average man. The other differences between these two products are the sodium and the carbohydrate content, both of which are slightly higher in the light version. Neither product is a significant source of vitamins or minerals.

Light Mayonnaise

2 tablespoons

Nutrition Facts

Serving Size (30g)
Servings Per Container

Amount Per Serving

Calories 100   Calories from Fat 90

% Daily Value*

Total Fat 10g	**15%**
Saturated Fat 1.5g	**8%**
Trans Fat 0g	
Cholesterol 10mg	**3%**
Sodium 240mg	**10%**
Total Carbohydrate 3g	**1%**
Dietary Fiber 0g	**0%**
Sugars 1g	
Protein 0g	

Vitamin A 2%   •   Vitamin C 0%

Calcium 0%   •   Iron 0%

*Percent Daily Values are based on a 2,000 calorie diet. Your daily values may be higher or lower depending on your calorie needs:

		Calories:	2,000	2,500
Total Fat	Less than		65g	80g
Saturated Fat	Less than		20g	25g
Cholesterol	Less than		300mg	300mg
Sodium	Less than		2,400mg	2,400mg
Total Carbohydrate			300g	375g
Dietary Fiber			25g	30g

Calories per gram:
Fat 9 • Carbohydrate 4 • Protein 4

Regular Mayonnaise

2 tablespoons

Nutrition Facts

Serving Size (28g)
Servings Per Container

Amount Per Serving

Calories 200   Calories from Fat 200

% Daily Value*

Total Fat 22g	**34%**
Saturated Fat 3g	**15%**
Trans Fat 0g	
Cholesterol 10mg	**3%**
Sodium 150mg	**6%**
Total Carbohydrate 0g	**0%**
Dietary Fiber 0g	**0%**
Sugars 0g	
Protein 0g	

Vitamin A 0%   •   Vitamin C 0%

Calcium 0%   •   Iron 0%

*Percent Daily Values are based on a 2,000 calorie diet. Your daily values may be higher or lower depending on your calorie needs:

		Calories:	2,000	2,500
Total Fat	Less than		65g	80g
Saturated Fat	Less than		20g	25g
Cholesterol	Less than		300mg	300mg
Sodium	Less than		2,400mg	2,400mg
Total Carbohydrate			300g	375g
Dietary Fiber			25g	30g

Calories per gram:
Fat 9 • Carbohydrate 4 • Protein 4

Don't Be Misled by Portion Sizes

One morning a young couple and their four-year-old son appeared in my office because their child's weight (compared to his height) was off the charts when he was weighed at his pediatrician's office during a routine visit. The parents were obviously worried about their overweight child and wanted to know what to do. Both parents were within their normal weight range and seemed to like a wide range of healthy food. They told me that they were trying to serve their son foods according to the portions on the nutrition facts on packages. Now you know that the nutrition facts are based on a 2000-Calorie intake and the portion size is determined solely by the food manufacturer.

So these parents were actually serving their four-year-old double the calories that he actually needed in an average day (approximately 1000 Calories). And he had become accustomed to eating portions that were similar to what his parents consumed. Once they learned that their child's portions could be less than the portions listed on packages, they were able to slowly taper the amounts they were feeding their child, giving him a chance to adjust gradually to less than he was accustomed to eating. He is gradually growing in height without gaining weight rather than being on a weight reduction diet.

This example provides an important lesson in reading labels and knowing each person's needs. Food portions are presented simply to illustrate what is contained in a specific serving size of the food. That does not mean that it's the portion we actually eat or that this portion is what our body needs at this time. Eating that does not include awareness of our own hunger and fullness levels, as well as our nutritional needs, can lead us astray. Never let a package dictate how much you need to eat.

Whole-Grain Labels

"Your threshing will continue until grape harvest and the grape harvest will continue until planting, and you will eat all the food you want and live in safety in your land."
—Leviticus 26:5

Not all whole-grain products are labeled with a Whole Grain Stamp, which was developed by the Whole Grains Council in 2005 to assist consumers. You can check the list of ingredients to see if the product is made with whole grains. Multigrain products simply tell you that the food product is made with many grains, which doesn't mean they are whole grains. A whole-grain product, however, may contain a variety of grains such as whole-wheat flour, whole-rye flour, and whole-grain cornmeal. And some whole-grain products can be very refined. Look at the texture difference between old-fashioned oatmeal and the typical O-shaped cold cereal made with oat flour. The less refined the grain, the better.

When you do see a stamp it's important to know that here are two types of Whole Grain stamps on food products. The 100% Whole Grain Stamp indicates that all of the grain ingredients are whole grains—a full serving is considered at least 16 grams. The Basic Stamp indicates that the product contains at least 8 grams (or ½ serving) of whole grains, but it might also contain some more refined grains or added fiber (bran) or added germ (such as wheat germ) that is not part of the whole grain ingredients. A whole grain is an intact grain that contains all 3 parts—bran, germ, and endosperm.

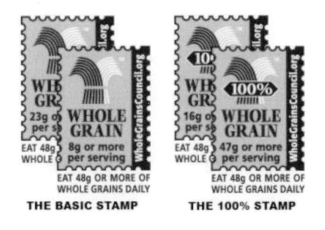

THE BASIC STAMP   **THE 100% STAMP**

Courtesy Oldways and the Whole Grains Council, www.wholegrainscouncil.org

Each stamp also shows a number, telling you how many grams of whole grain ingredients are in a serving of the product. So it's easier to tell if you are getting 3 servings of whole grains per day (a total of 48 grams), when you eat several foods that add up to the 48 grams. Some products that have the Basic Stamp simply state "Good Source" so you can assume that a serving provides you with 8 grams of whole grain.

In the first chapter I advised you to make half the grains you eat whole grains. But are 3 servings really enough if you eat a diet that contains more than 2000 Calories per day? If you do a lot of physical work or exercise and you're consuming 8 or 10 servings of grains per day, then you should make half of them (4–5) whole grains. And if you are on a low-carbohydrate diet and eat only 3 servings of grain or starch per day, should they all be whole grains? The answer ideally is yes. The bottom line advice is to consume as many whole grains as possible, but at least 3 a day, or a total of 48 grams, as part of a healthy diet.

What to Do When There's No Label

Nutrition labels are rarely found when you're shopping for fresh items such as fish, meat, fruits, and vegetables. These can be among the healthiest foods in the market, but how do you compare the nutrition value of what you see? Some markets provide a printed reference with facts about foods that don't come packaged with labels. For instance, some produce departments have reference books or cards that describe all of the varieties of produce that they carry. This information may include nutrient content, purchasing and storage information, and photos to help you identify the items on display.

Aliza Green's *Field Guide* series provides helpful pocketsize volumes on produce, seafood, and herbs and spices that can be easily taken to the grocery store or used at home for reference. These books give useful tips on how to tell if an item is ripe and even includes basic cooking techniques for the foods listed. A paperback book such as Corinne Netzer's *Complete Book of Food Counts* contains details such as the fat content of various cuts of meat and the potassium content of different fruits and vegetables. (See the Resources section on p. 183.) If you are on a special medical diet you might need this level of detail.

When selecting meats, generally the expensive prime cuts contain the highest amount of fat and the choice or good cuts are usually leaner. Look at the meat to see how much visible fat is present in the package. For instance, if most of the fat is on the outside of a pork chop you will be able to trim it easily before cooking, but if a rib steak has extensive marbling of the fat throughout, you will not be able to remove most of the fat and not all of it will drip off during cooking.

One of the questions I'm asked most often is whether to buy organic produce. Since there is not yet scientific evidence that pesticides may be implicated in cancer and other health problems, you may want to know when to spend the extra money for "organic" or "pesticide-free" fruits and vegetables. The Environmental Working Group has published a list of the most and least pesticide-contaminated fruits and vegetables. This may help you decide when to spend the extra money to avoid the greatest amount of pesticides. And buying locally in season can help to keep the cost of produce down while giving you a better chance of finding foods that aren't so chemically treated, even if they're not certified as organic. Keep in mind that organic produce may cost two to three times as much as regular produce, so if you're on a limited budget the best choice may be to buy non-organic items, wash them thoroughly and peel any thick skins. Your first priority should be getting enough fruits and vegetables to eat within the food budget you have.

The "Clean 15" have the least pesticide residue:

Asparagus	Mango
Avocado	Onion
Broccoli	Papaya
Cabbage	Pineapple
Corn	Sweet potato
Eggplant	Tomato
Green peas	Watermelon
Kiwi	

The "Dirty Dozen" have the most pesticide residue:

Apple	Kale
Bell pepper	Lettuce
Carrot	Nectarine
Celery	Peach
Cherries	Pear
Imported grapes	Strawberries

Don't hesitate to ask the vendors at your local farmers' markets about their growing practices. Sometimes I buy the local produce that isn't organic if it's very fresh. It has a lower carbon footprint if it hasn't had to travel across the world, and the price is lower.

Tips for Smart Shopping

Before making out the grocery list take an inventory of what you need and what staple food items you may want to replenish if they are on sale.

Keep a running list of what you need posted on the refrigerator and add to it as you run out of items or think of things you'll need (ask everyone in your household to do this).

Open the refrigerator as you're preparing breakfast or starting your day to see if there are items that you need to replenish soon.

Transport your food safely from the market to your home. Utilize the inexpensive, reusable insulated totes that may be available at your grocery store. Don't leave perishable items in the trunk of your car unless the outside temperature is below 38 degrees. Consider keeping a cooler in the trunk of your car in warm weather. Simply pop in some ice packs when you go shopping and refreeze them when you unpack your groceries—you'll be ready for the next shopping trip.

Before buying, check expiration dates on dairy products, perishables, and packaged items such as whole grain breads to get the maximum shelf life once you take the food home.

Don't be fooled by health claims on the front of packaged foods. Turn the package over and look at the ingredient list and the nutrition facts label before you put an item in your grocery cart. Make up your own mind about which foods are healthy for you.

Keeping Good Food Fresh, Safe, and Ready

Food is for eating, and good food is to be enjoyed. . . .
I think food is, actually, very beautiful in itself.
—Delia Smith, CBE (1941–)

I T'S NO WONDER THAT FOR HUNDREDS OF YEARS artists have used real food as the subject of their still life paintings. What is more attractive than a beautiful bowl of fruit on the kitchen table? And storing good food in plain sight reminds us not only of its beauty but also of its availability. Most food requires more preparation to store it than an apple or pear that is washed, dried, and placed in the fruit bowl.

The beauty of real food can add a touch of divine beauty to your kitchen counter or your refrigerator. Consider a bowl of fruit a source of inspiration, reminding us of these beautiful gifts of whole food that can help us to live a whole life—mind, body, and spirit.

> The beauty of real food can add a touch of divine beauty to your kitchen counter or your refrigerator.

I've always coveted one of those refrigerators that have a full-length glass door. I would love to see the colors of the produce right through the door, but what I do like is to open the doors of my traditional refrigerator and see the food stored in glass containers or clear storage bags.

Healthy food should be as accessible for eating as quick junk food. Having basic fruits, vegetables, whole grains, and lean proteins available takes some planning and advance preparation. At first it may seem to require a lot of work and attention, but with practice you'll get the hang of it.

We can take a lesson from restaurant chefs and how they organize meal preparation in advance. When you are seated in a restaurant and place your order, do you really think the chef starts peeling the carrots and washing the lettuce then? Of course not! When the cooking staff arrives earlier in the day, they peel the carrots, marinate the chicken, wash and peel the vegetables, and make the desserts and breads. Some of the preparation of the ingredients is done even earlier in the week when the food delivery arrives. For example, heads of lettuce may be trimmed of bruised spots, washed, and crisped in the refrigerator.

Prepare your ingredients in advance for your meals at a time when you're not rushed or tired. Don't wait until you and your family get home after a busy day. It's more difficult to carry out your meal plan and prepare a simple recipe when you're hungry and tired. Now that you've done your meal planning and brought the groceries home, the next step is to store the food in a way that maximizes its shelf life and minimizes the work you have to do at mealtime.

Food preparation can begin when you bag items at the market together that will be stored together. Put all your items for the freezer in one bag. Most supermarkets now offer insulated reusable bags for frozen and perishable items. Even if it's the middle of winter and your frozen food will not thaw on your way home from the market, separating these items will save you time and steps when you get home. And it's a good habit to get into at any time of year.

On a hot summer day, consider placing a picnic cooler with ice packs in the trunk of your car to insure your food will be safe. Especially if small children, elderly folks, or pregnant women will be eating this food, prevent the risk of bacterial growth and food poisoning by keeping perishable food cold until you store it in your refrigerator or freezer.

When packing your purchases, designate one bag for items that will be prepped before storing when you get home. You might place all of the produce together in your shopping cart and then bag them together. When you get home, prep any fruits and vegetables that you will be using in the next three days. For instance, if your meal planning includes salad tomorrow, wash the lettuce or greens, spin them dry, and store in the refrigerator where they will be ready when you need them. Don't tear or cut the leaves into pieces yet, since that will encourage oxidation and browning, decreasing the shelf life and spoiling the appearance. And not all produce can be washed right away. For example, berries should be washed just before serving.

When you arrive home from the grocery store, place the groceries on the kitchen counter or table. Immediately store meat, fish, dairy, and other perishable items. This insures that those items will quickly return to less than 40 degrees and extends the shelf life by discouraging bacterial growth at 40–140 degrees (the temperature danger zone). Store your bananas, potatoes, and tomatoes at room temperature. Prepare ripe fruits such as pineapple or citrus fruit now. You can cut these fruits up and they will be ready to eat even if you're on the go. You can even make a fruit salad or fruit compote and portion it into small containers suitable for grab-and-go snacks or lunches. Sometimes it's easier to decide on the portion in advance of when you will eat it, but stay conscious of your hunger and fullness level when you are actually eating.

Wash all fruits that will be placed in a fruit bowl—for example, an assortment of apples, plums, pears, and grapes. Put the bowl out in a central place where it will give the visual cue to eat something healthy that is fresh and ready when you or your family are hungry.

You'll find that prepping your food in advance will save you time and reduce your stress at mealtime. When you wash, peel, and cut foods at one time you'll also reduce the number of times you open and close the refrigerator, saving energy. And you'll only have to wash your prep utensils once. You're also more likely to carry out your meal plan and prepare the recipes you've chosen, including all of the fruits and vegetables you've bought. Less food will be discarded as it sits untouched in the refrigerator.

> You'll find that prepping your food in advance will save you time and reduce your stress at mealtime.

As you are preparing food for storage or for preparation for a meal in the future, be conscious, too, of food safety. Always wash and prepare your fruit, vegetables, dairy, and other foods that will not be cooked before handling meats, fish, or eggs in the kitchen. So, if you decide to cut up a whole chicken and freeze part of it for another day, wait until all of your fresh groceries have been processed and stored. Even if you're slicing vegetables for a chicken stir-fry tomorrow, cut the vegetables first and store them separately from the chicken. This reduces the possibility of contamination of raw foods with bacteria from the meat.

Food Safety Musts

Even the most beautiful, delicious, and nutritious food can be unhealthy if it's not stored and handled safely.

- Store food in the refrigerator or freezer immediately after shopping or finishing a meal. Never leave food out on the counter any longer than necessary.

- Store eggs in their carton, not on the door of the refrigerator where the temperature is warmer. The carton will help prevent the eggs from absorbing food odors.

- When in doubt, throw it out. If a food tastes or smells suspicious, discard it.

- Never store food and cleaning products or chemicals in the same area.

- Keep perishable food out of the temperature danger zone (40–140 degrees) as much as possible. Store dry ingredients and staples such as pasta at 50–70 degrees if possible.

- Get into the habit of checking food temperatures with an instant-read thermometer to make sure they have cooked or cooled to the proper temperature.

- Wash your hands often when cooking, and don't forget to clean faucet, utensil, and appliance handles, which may become contaminated with bacteria from food.

- Avoid cross-contamination of raw foods and meats by using separate cutting boards for each and sanitizing the boards by washing in the dishwasher or by hand with a mixture of bleach and water.

When you start your food prep and begin putting foods away, there are many choices for food storage containers available today. I have a variety of containers, from the set of Pyrex® glass containers and lids that I received as a wedding present, to newer plastic containers that are designed to extend the shelf life of salad greens or berries. I prefer clear glass, Lexan, or plastic because of the visibility of the food within. Sometimes I use a zip-type 1-gallon bag when storing the vegetables that I've prepared for making a recipe such as Roasted Summer Vegetables. These fit nicely into the vegetable bin and don't take up a lot of space, but I don't recommend reusing them. Plastic food-storage bags or bottles are considered safe for a single use but should not used again even if they are washed, since they are porous and can harbor harmful bacteria. Never reuse plastic food packages such as cottage cheese or yogurt containers for the same reason. You can still reuse plastic bags or bottles in other environmentally friendly ways, but not for food-related use.

Washable glass or clear plastic food-grade containers cost more to buy but can be reused again and again. One reason I prefer nonreactive glass or ceramic containers is that I can also take them from refrigerator to freezer to microwave or oven. And I only use nonreactive containers when microwaving frozen vegetables. Generally I buy frozen items that come packaged in paper rather than plastic, and I never microwave anything in plastic packages or containers. Nonreactive containers and packages that are labeled "safe for microwave use" are less likely to interact with the food causing harmful chemicals to migrate into the food.

If you do microwave using plastic wrap, don't let the plastic touch foods during cooking. Leave at least an inch between the wrap and the food surface. Better yet, buy a domed plastic lid that can be placed over a container of food in the microwave. It's washable and reusable and will not come into direct contact with the food.

Advance preparation not only involves preparing raw ingredients for meals, but it also encompasses storing portions of meals for future use. These "planned-overs" or make-ahead meals or side dishes can consolidate your cooking time and be a healthier and less expensive alternative to take-out meals on a busy day. I recommend storing extra portions of meals before sitting down to dinner. There is less chance of overeating if extra foods are stored before dinner begins. Designate in advance any foods that will be refrigerated or frozen for future use. Even small portions of leftover meats, starches, or vegetables can be frozen in small bags or containers and added to a soup or casserole later. And how great it is to enjoy a home-cooked, lovingly prepared meal the next day for lunch, or even next month after a hectic day when there's been no time for cooking.

Storing foods properly can extend the shelf life and reduce food dollars that end up in the trash or the compost pile. Labeling and dating are a vital habit in kitchen economics. A few minutes spent with a waterproof pen and some labels pay big dividends. Let your children get involved and they will learn a practical conservation lesson.

Storage Guidelines for Good Food

To achieve the longest storage life for your foods, always check the "sell-by," "use-by," "expiration," or "freshness" date on the package. Some food items that have a long shelf life such as pasta or frozen entrées are marked with a "best if used by" date. These foods are apt to lose quality but can be safely used for a short time after that date. Canned or jarred foods such as fruit, vegetables, and tomato sauce can be used up to one year from the date they are packaged.

Frozen fruits and vegetables can be stored in the freezer for six to eight months but often taste better if used sooner. Fresh apples can be stored for up to a month in the refrigerator, and grapefruit and oranges can be stored for about two weeks before losing moisture, flavor, and vitamins. Other fresh fruit needs to be ripened and can be stored for a few days in the refrigerator, but check daily for freshness.

Fresh vegetables such as summer squashes, peppers, and greens can be refrigerated for three to five days. Root vegetables, winter squashes, onions, and potatoes should be stored in a cool place with adequate ventilation to prevent spoilage, but never in the refrigerator. I find that my basement or a cool storage cabinet is closest to the 50-60 degree temperature that is ideal.

Dairy products are among the most perishable foods. Pay attention to the date on the container when buying milk and don't leave it at room temperature; just pour it and store it. If stored properly, opened containers of milk can be kept in the refrigerator for up to one week. Boxed milk is shelf stable at room temperature but should be refrigerated after opening the package. Cheese of any kind should be stored in the refrigerator. Once it is opened you should wrap the cheese to prevent moisture loss. You can safely remove any mold that develops on hard cheese by cutting it off with a knife, but discard soft cheese, cottage cheese, or dairy sour cream that shows any discoloration or signs of mold.

Meat, poultry, eggs, and fish are not only very perishable but also have the potential for causing food poisoning if not stored properly and used promptly. Ideally you should use meat and poultry within three days of purchase. Otherwise freeze it until

A Lesson in Managing Waste

Early in my career I learned many lessons in preventing waste and utilizing ingredients that might otherwise be discarded. These were not lessons learned in school but from a frugal man who ran the bakeshop in the hospital where I worked as a college student. Bill had left his native Germany at the age of twelve to apprentice on a ship as a cook. He had been kneading dough for so many years that his fingertips had a permanently upturned shape. Bill would start every morning at 5 AM by wandering through the main kitchen to see what ingredients he might use that day to enhance his baked goods.

This made for interesting and delicious banana bran muffins and zucchini cakes. He would not waste a crumb. After baking cookies and removing the cookies from the baking sheets to cool on racks, Bill would scrape the remaining crumbs and pieces of broken cookies into large airtight tins so that he could include these morsels in future creations. It's no wonder he was so skilled at keeping within the budget without sacrificing taste. Bill might be amused today if he could hear us comment on his green practices, but we can all take a cue from his thoughtful approach to cooking.

needed. Fish should be used within one to two days of buying it. Eggs can be kept for about a month in the carton in the refrigerator, but the quality will be the best if they are used sooner. You can hard-boil eggs and store them for an additional week in the refrigerator.

Five Ways to Prevent Food Waste and Spoilage

- Freeze items that are used infrequently to prolong shelf life, such as nuts and whole-grain flour. These are not as perishable as produce but will lose flavor and nutrients and become rancid when stored for long periods of time at room temperature, especially in hot, humid weather.
- Check your food inventory before you make out your grocery list to avoid having food on the shelf for extended periods of time, as this decreases flavor and quality.

- **Store** raw meat or fish on the bottom shelf of your refrigerator to avoid cross-contamination with other foods such as fruit and vegetables.

- **Thaw** foods in the refrigerator or microwave, never at room temperature, to minimize the time they spend in the temperature danger zone (40–140 degrees) where bacterial growth is more rapid.

- **Keep** labels and waterproof markers handy near your food prep area and storage supplies. Label and date everything as you store it.

Making Good Food Taste Great

You don't have to cook fancy or complicated masterpieces, just good food from fresh ingredients.

—Julia Child (1912–2004)

C OOKING SKILL COVERS A WIDE RANGE OF ABILITY, from reheating frozen meals in a microwave to sophisticated gourmet creations. Although culinary skills don't guarantee eating right, they do make it easier to cook a wide variety of whole foods and to plan meals that will be appealing as well as healthy.

I grew up eating my mother's cooking, good wholesome food seasoned with butter, salt, and pepper. Nothing exotic. But I learned the basics of producing a healthy meal and the skills involved in making all the items in the meal finish at the same time. I always looked forward to holidays because I knew my father would be cooking, and that meant some spices and herbs would be added to the turkey or the roast and some creativity was infused into every meal.

Fortunately, I grew up in an Italian neighborhood in Boston and developed a taste for Mediterranean food at an early age. I learned cooking techniques from friends and from my grandparents. As the oldest child in a family of seven children, I volunteered to cook family dinners from the time I was about sixteen. I was motivated to learn more about cooking so that I could enjoy great-tasting food myself. My brothers did not always appreciate my experimenting with their favorite dishes, but even their occasional complaints did not deter me from mastering my cooking skills. I became a fan of Julia Child from her first episode on television and an avid reader of innovative nutritionist Adelle Davis's books, such as *Let's Eat Right to Keep Fit*. I like to think that I have blended the best of what I have learned from both of these pioneers in cooking and health.

I believe that cooking skill involves being motivated to produce the finished product, whether an apple pie or some homemade pasta. The ability to read is essential, as is some basic hand-eye coordination. And if you are willing to make mistakes, there is hope that you can master basic cooking and perhaps even more complicated recipes. Adult education classes that feature cooking instruction and hands-on experience are available in almost every county across the country. Now even some restaurants give cooking demonstrations or classes with a chef. And the Food Network features television programs such as *Healthy Appetite* with registered dietitian Ellie Krieger that can help to improve your cooking skills and your knowledge of good nutrition.

Whatever you do, start with small steps to prepare good food in your own kitchen. Begin with some of your favorite recipes and see how you can make them even healthier. Try some of the seasoning suggestions and ideas for garnishing that follow in this chapter. Be brave and try a new herb or an entirely new cuisine. Sample some of the recipes in chapter 12 and be prepared to enjoy good food in your life every day. Making small changes to let your mind, body and spirit adjust gradually will not involve sweeping overnight changes, but small steps will lead to big results over time.

> Start with small steps to prepare good food in your own kitchen. Begin with some of your favorite recipes and see how you can make them even healthier.

Tips for Making Your Favorite Recipes Healthier

- Cut pasta amounts in half while doubling the vegetables in recipes.
- Cut the amount of salad dressing or marinade in half or dilute it with water.
- Rinse salty foods such as olives, canned beets, beans, and capers before using to reduce the sodium content.
- Instead of using a tablespoon of butter to brown meat or fish, sauté with a combination of butter and olive oil (put ½ teaspoon butter in a tablespoon and fill up the measuring spoon with olive oil). This will give you more monounsaturated plant fat (healthy fat) and less saturated animal fat, making your dish healthier. You will still taste the butter in the finished product.
- Use nonfat buttermilk or nonfat Greek yogurt in place of cream in soups, salad dressings, and desserts whenever possible to reduce unhealthy saturated fat.
- When ordering pizza, ask for "half cheese" and "double cut" to reduce calories and make it easier to choose a small slice

Seasoning Methods

Even if you've always thought that the use of seasonings was too complex, some simple seasoning methods can add flavor and appeal to vegetables, fruits, whole grains, and other foods you are trying to include in your daily diet. Even simple foods can be presented creatively and artfully with relatively little effort. Start to think of your plate as an artist's palette; add color and flavor at the same time. Add small amounts of seasonings and then taste. You can always add more later.

download this chart online at
www.3DYourWholeLife.com!

Seasoning	Uses
Allspice	Meats, fruit desserts
Anise seed	Chicken, baked goods, breads
Basil, fresh	Tomato, eggplant, salads, Asian foods, pesto
Basil, dried	Tomato sauces, cooked vegetables, soups, stews
Bay leaves	Soups, stews, tomato sauce, dried beans
Caraway seed	European, Asian, Indian food, cabbage, baked goods, bread
Cardamom, pods or ground	Stews, curries, baked goods
Cayenne pepper	Heats up any type of savory food or sauce
Celery seed	Soups, sauces, cole slaw, dressings
Chervil	Eggs, salads, soups, chicken
Chives	Fish, meat, vegetables, sauces, soups, eggs
Cilantro, sweet or hot	Asian, Spanish, Southwestern food, pesto
Cinnamon, ground or sticks	Baked goods, fruit desserts, stews, curries
Cloves, whole or ground	Baked goods, stews, curries, pork
Coriander	Baked goods, curries, Indian food
Cumin	Soups, stews, chili, Mexican/Southwestern food
Curry powder	Curries, seafood, vegetables, soups
Dill and dill seed	Fish, eggs, vegetables, baked goods, sauces

Fennel seed	Sauces, stews, pork
Garlic powder	Use when fresh garlic is not available
Ginger, ground	Baked goods, Asian food
Juniper berries	Meat, game, stews
Lavender flowers, stems, leaves	Salads, desserts, baked goods
Lemon grass	Asian food, seafood, vegetables
Mace	Custards, baked goods, fruit desserts
Marjoram	Soups, stews
Mint	Garnish fruit, chicken, salads
Mustard seed, whole or ground	Meat, sauces
Nutmeg, whole or ground	Baked goods, fruit desserts, cheese sauces, soups
Onion powder or flakes	Use when fresh onion not available
Oregano	Pizza, chili, soups, vegetables, tomato sauces
Paprika, hot or sweet	Hungarian food, deviled eggs, soups, poultry, fish, and garnish
Parsley, curly or flat-leaf	Universal garnish, soups, stews, sauces, entrées
Peppercorns, all colors	Universal seasoning, whole or ground
Poppy seeds, black or white	Baked goods, salad dressings, noodles
Red pepper flakes	Heats or intensifies the flavor of savory foods
Rosemary	Fish, lamb, chicken, shrimp, sauces, baked goods
Saffron	Soups, curries, risotto, rice
Sage	Beef, pork, chicken, stews, winter squash, stuffing
Sesame Seeds, black or white	Baked goods, salmon, salads, vegetables, stir-fry
Savory, winter or summer	Soups, meats, fish, beans
Tarragon	Chicken, fish, eggs, sauces, salad dressings
Thyme, many varieties	Eggs, soups, poultry, fish, vegetables
Turmeric	Curries, stews
Vanilla pods or extract	Baked goods, custards, desserts
Wasabi, ground horseradish	Heats and adds color to sauces, fish, meat, Asian food

Seasoning Blends

These blends can save time by combining common mixtures of seasonings and are available in most grocery stores or in specialty food stores. The package labels give suggestions for use in specific types of foods. Or experiment by sprinkling a dash on an omelet, a baked potato, or a plain meat or fish portion.

Cajun spice

Chili powder

Chinese five-spice powder

Garam masala

Greek seasoning

Herbes de Provence

Italian seasoning

Lemon pepper

Mrs. Dash® seasonings

McCormick® salt-free seasoning blends

Old Bay® seasoning

Pumpkin pie spice

Taco seasoning

Other Seasonings and Flavor Enhancers

Anchovies and anchovy paste

Capers

Citrus zest and juices

Garlic

Green peppercorns, fresh or brined

Horseradish, fresh or prepared

Onion

Shallots

Getting the Best of Spices and Herbs

The shelf life of dried herbs and spices depends on whether they are stored in their whole form, such as whole cloves, leaf thyme, or cardamom pods, or whether they are ground. In general tightly sealed glass jars of whole dried herbs will last one to two years on your shelf if they are stored away from heat, light, and moisture.

If the spices or herbs are ground, they will lose flavor more quickly and should be replaced every six months. An easy way to keep track of your spices' freshness is to write the date you first opened the jar with an indelible marker on the side of the container.

Tried-and-True Seasoning Combinations

These tried-and-true seasoning combinations add flavor, nutrients, and fragrance to foods such as soups, stews, roasts, and vegetables.

"The Holy Trinity"
onion, celery, and carrots

"The Four Evangelists"
onion, celery, carrots, and garlic

To get the best flavor from your dried herbs, crush them in your hand before adding them to food to release the natural oils.

From Beige to Beautiful: The Value of Garnishes

A beautiful plate satisfies the visual appetite as well as the physical. Try to select garnishes that contribute some nutrient content without adding excessive calories. A plain tuna salad sandwich on your plate will look more appetizing if you add a cluster of a dozen grapes or a wedge of melon. And you and your family are more likely to include fruit in the meal if it's on the main plate. A couple of sprigs of parsley will add color, flavor, and nutrients to a dinner plate, and they will provide a small but significant amount of vitamin A, beta carotene, and potassium in less than 1 Calorie. Besides, parsley is a time-honored breath freshener.

Nearly every chronic disease that develops as we age can be prevented or delayed by a greater intake of fruits, vegetables, and other highly pigmented foods.

Beyond the vitamin and mineral contribution of edible garnishes is their content of antioxidants. Nearly every chronic disease that develops as we age can be prevented or delayed by a greater intake of fruits, vegetables, and other highly pigmented foods.

And garnishes can add interest and make a food more appealing. For example, using a favorite garnish may make a new food more enticing. Or including crunchy cucumbers with a sandwich can satisfy the need for crunch that potato chips provide, without the excess calories.

Garnishes: Dress Up for Dinner

- Lemons, limes: wedges, slices, or twisted slices (cut half way across lemon slices and twist the ends in opposite directions)
- Orange crowns: using a whole orange and a small paring knife, cut each orange around the middle using a saw-tooth pattern. Each half looks like a crown.
- Tomato: slices, wedges, small whole grape or cherry tomatoes
- Cucumber: slices, spears, cubes, with or without skin
- Carrot: coins, diagonal slices, sticks, shredded
- Melon: slices, wedges, balls
- Strawberries: fans (slice berries lengthwise from the tip almost all the way toward the top, then fan out slices on the plate)
- Pepper: rings, matchsticks, cookie cutter shapes
- Green onion: sliced or brushes (slice off roots and dark green portion on top. Cut slashes at both ends of the onion to resemble fringe. Soak for a few minutes in a bowl of ice water to curl the ends to look like brushes)
- Herb sprigs (parsley, cilantro, basil, chives, watercress)
- Lettuce, spinach, kale: use alone as a base for food items or as an under layer for other garnishes
- Ketchup, mustard, sauces: using a ladle, a squeeze bottle, or a plastic bag with a small hole cut in one corner, drizzle in Z pattern or dots on the food or around the rim of the plate

Tips for Making the Most of Seasonings

▪ Try a new spice or herb each week to increase your repertoire of flavors and their contribution of antioxidants, vitamins, and minerals.

▪ Keep dried or frozen herbs available when fresh herbs are not in season or are too expensive.

▪ Buy spices and herbs in the smallest quantities available—this is one item that you don't want to buy in bulk. They will lose flavor over time so larger amounts would be wasted.

▪ Measure spices and herbs in advance, away from the stove. Never shake a spice directly from the bottle or jar over a steaming pot of food, since the moisture will affect the spice when recapped and stored, and it will shorten the shelf life.

▪ Garnish to add beauty and valuable nutrients to even the humblest food.

Cooking Methods

I think I was the last person I know who bought a microwave oven. Since I enjoy cooking so much I didn't see the need for cooking things in a rush. But now I wouldn't want to be without it. I use it for everyday jobs like defrosting meats, cooking vegetables, melting chocolate, and reheating foods. I even have one in my office just for heating up soup for lunch or making a quick cup of tea. Studies show that 95 percent of U.S. households now have a microwave.

Microwave cooking has its advantages. It is energy efficient; it uses 30–70 percent less energy than boiling on the top of the stove or roasting foods in the oven. It is quicker, since many items cook in one-quarter the time in the microwave. That may mean that you would be more likely to include a cooked vegetable in a quick meal. Microwaving retains more nutrients in foods such as vegetables, because cooking time is shorter and less water needs to be added. Colors stay truer and more appealing. And it's not necessary to add salt or fat to cook. There is also less clean-up necessary. Who minds fewer pots to wash?

Reheat Safely

Leftovers should always be reheated to a temperature of 165 degrees. If you microwave to reheat, let the food stand for 2 minutes after cooking to complete the reheating and to reach the maximum temperature. Use an instant-read thermometer to check the temperature.

Stovetop cooking can be more energy-efficient than cooking food in the oven. It allows you to sear and brown a food. My favorite for this task is the black cast iron skillet, which I mentioned earlier when describing essential cooking equipment.

Grilling can be a fun way to cook during warm summer months, or it may be a way to get other family members involved in the cooking. And some foods just taste better grilled. Smoke, spills, and smells stay outside and not in your kitchen. More fat may drip off foods such as meat and marinated items, but avoid charring meats and fish. Turn often, because unhealthy (potentially cancer-causing) compounds can be produced in animal protein cooked over a flame at high heat.

Easy Peeling with the Help of Your Microwave

- To peel onions, place them on a covered microwave-safe plate and cook for 1 to 2 minutes at full power.
- To peel a head of garlic, remove the outer papery skin from garlic cloves, place them in a custard cup, and microwave at 80 percent power for 30 seconds. Allow the cloves to cool enough so you can handle them and then lift away the skin.

Try indirect cooking on the grill for a change. Brown the meat gently over the flame, then move to the non-flame side of the grill and close the cover to continue to cook slowly, thereby keeping the meat moister.

Slow cooking may help you to cut down on take-out meals. You can assemble the ingredients the night before and refrigerate. The next day simply combine the ingredients in your slow cooker and plug it in before you leave for the day. All you have to do is dish it up to enjoy this healthy kind of convenience food.

Traditional cooking methods such as baking can be varied by using equipment such as tagine pots or clay ovens for cooking meat dishes. Broiling is a convenient way to quickly cook fish or meat, allowing fat to drip off during the cooking. Countertop rotisserie cookers are also great for cooking meats, since they also allow fat to drip off during the cooking process and yet keep the meat very moist. Electric skillets can also be a handy addition to your appliances, since they can free up stovetop burners or the oven when you are cooking for a crowd. And variety in your cooking techniques will produce a variety of flavors and textures that will keep your meals interesting.

SHARING

Where and How Do You Eat?

Do you eat alone or with others most of the time?

Do you eat sitting or do you eat standing, walking, driving?

Do you play background music or watch television while eating?

Do you read during meals?

Do you answer phone calls during dinner?

Do you say grace or privately give thanks before meals,
or do you just dig in?

Do you eat dinner in <10 minutes or >30 minutes?

Do you eat lunch in <10 minutes or >20 minutes?

WHICH OF THESE HABITS COULD YOU PLAN TO IMPROVE TODAY?

The Sacred Table
Where and How You Eat

On that day HOLY TO THE LORD will be inscribed on the bells
of the horses, and the cooking pots in the LORD'S house
will be like the sacred bowls in front of the altar.
—Zechariah 14:19–21

I GREW UP WITH THE TEACHING that our bodies are temples of the Holy Spirit and as such we should respect and care for them in the best way possible. And so not only is the kind of food we use to nourish our bodies important, but also the way we partake of those meals. Now that you are planning what to eat to meet your nutritional needs and preparing meals that are appealing, it is time to turn your attention to how and where you consume those meals.

When considering what makes a meal sacred, our first association may be with an Easter or Christmas dinner, celebrating a religious holiday after a period of fasting or a wedding feast. But a sacred meal may also be one in which we volunteer at a soup kitchen or work with others in our church to prepare a meal for the needy in the community. Or it can be a meal that is brought to us by a friend when we are in need. I think that meals are always sacred if we make them so—not just by cooking a feast for Thanksgiving but every day we enjoy a meal with thanks to God in our hearts for the food we eat, the body we are nourishing, and the company of those at our table with whom we are breaking bread. Fast food eaten mindlessly without thought or thanks would be anything but blessed.

I am constantly inspired by my clients and patients who struggle with acute and chronic illness and yet manage to be grateful for the foods they can eat and the healing they feel when they eat right. To me something sacred is so important that it's worthy of my time, my respect, and my full attention.

I consider my calling as a nutritionist a sacred one, but I am also dedicated to seeing that my family has healthy meals and that we share them together at our table at least once a day. I also think that the dinner table is a great equalizer in the sense that we all come to the table as equals, hungry souls looking for nourishment, no matter who we are or what our status in life.

One of the first things to attend to in eating attentively and gratefully is paying attention to where we eat. Decide on designated eating areas in home and in your workplace. At home you might utilize the obvious areas of the kitchen, the dining room, at a table in the backyard, or a spot on the porch. If we nibble while standing at the counter or at the refrigerator with the door open, or munch something mindlessly while sitting at a computer, we aren't paying attention and it doesn't even register in our brains or in our stomachs.

Avoid multitasking while eating—for instance, working on the computer and eating lunch, watching the evening news while eating dinner, eating breakfast while driving your car. Actually setting time aside to eat and look at your food can help to enhance your satiety. You will increase your satisfaction with meals when you focus on what you are doing. Of course there are cultural exceptions, like snacking while watching the Super Bowl!

> Make each dinner a time of celebration and enjoyment with each other even if it's leftover meatloaf and carrots.

The Family Dinner

Not only is it important to pay attention to *what* and *where* we eat, making every day meals nourishing for your body, but *how* we eat can be an opportunity to nourish the spirit as well. Make each dinner a time of celebration and enjoyment with each other even if it's leftover meatloaf and carrots. Share not only your food but the details of your day. Sitting down to a family dinner is what knits the yarns of each individual's life together into a family fabric. In years to come, you may not remember the take-out pizza that was consumed in front of the television set, but you will remember the enjoyment of nourishing meals, eaten in a leisurely manner, with good conversation in the company of family and friends. Even a task as menial as doing the dishes after a good meal can have a sacramental importance to it. To rush is to miss these important spiritual aspects.

As a member of a large family, I became accustomed early in life to eating and serving family-style meals. Sometimes everything would be served at the table, and sometimes my mother would plate the entrée and vegetables for us and we could help ourselves to bread and butter, applesauce, or other side dishes at the table. At other times the food would be plated from the stove or the counter, but we always sat down together and had a family meal. Even my earliest restaurant meals in the fabled dining rooms at the Durgin Park Restaurant in Boston were taken in a family-style atmosphere. The tables for the clientele were long and parties sat together. The waitresses would enlist the help of the guests as needed to pass food or clear the tables. People from all over the world still go to have dinner at Durgin Park because of the traditional New England food and the ambience of the family dinner table.

Pros and Cons of Family-style Meals

PROS

- Everyone can choose their own portion
- Individuals can select only those items they choose to eat
- Less food is wasted
- Increased interaction as dishes are passed around the table
- The cook can partake of the meal with everyone else

CONS

- Some may find it too tempting to have seconds
- It's harder to judge how much to cook
- There are extra serving dishes to wash
- Not everyone may taste every item served, especially children
- The cook doesn't have the opportunity to arrange the foods on the plate in a particular presentation

DOES FAMILY-STYLE MEAL SERVICE WORK FOR YOU?

Dinner for One

Sharing good food with family and friends is one of life's greatest joys, but that's not always possible if you live alone. That doesn't mean you can't enjoy good food as well as the nourishment and comfort one gets from a healthy and delicious meal that is well presented. You can still relax, refuel, and recharge when you put good food on the table.

Not everyone has the opportunity on a daily basis to eat meals with others. Your nest might be empty. You might be single or widowed and living alone. You might travel on business and have dinner by yourself in your hotel room. Dining alone does not prevent you from having a sacred mealtime experience.

Even if dinner is a frozen entrée, you can take it out of the package and put the contents on a nice plate. Microwave an extra vegetable to enhance the nutrition, appearance, and satisfaction you'll get from the meal. Or you might want to use the salad bar at the market to select a simple but well-balanced meal that is ready to take home and enjoy. You could choose cooked chicken or a hard-boiled egg and some chickpeas and a selection of vegetables such as greens, peppers, beets, radishes, or other raw vegetables.

Recipe websites like SparkRecipes.com and Cooks.com are great sources of inspiration and recipe ideas, with quantities adaptable for one person. I've listed more recipe websites in the Resources section at the end of the book. Just look for recipes that help you to include fruits, vegetables, healthy fats, and whole grains in your meals.

Planning and preparing are still essential steps to having good food even when it's not possible to share a meal with others. Eating right and living well can be fringe benefits when you're dining alone. And yes, you are worth the effort of doing this just for yourself!

Start with small steps to prepare good food in your own kitchen. Begin with some of your favorite recipes and see how you can make them even healthier.

Making Meals Matter

Whenever possible make meals a family or community affair. And make your table a loving place. A good meal can give physical form to your love of those you are serving. Treat yourself and your family and friends as you would most cherished guests. Meals can be the best time to share the day's experiences with those you love and can be a time of bonding among friends and family members. Ask each person at the table questions such as "What was the best moment of the day for you today?" If you live alone you might occasionally plan to eat with others during the day, whether it's meeting a friend for breakfast or coffee, planning to have lunch with a coworker in the cafeteria, or inviting someone over for dinner. Try not to eat alone all of the time. Reach out to others who would like company too. Eating communally can make us attentive to our eating and to enjoying food in a way that might not always be there when we eat alone.

Do not forget to entertain strangers, for by so doing
some people have entertained angels without knowing it.
—Hebrews 13:2

Never bring anger to the table if you can help it. Agree to disagree after the meal is over. And above all, don't call attention to others for eating or not eating something at the table. Some eating disorders can have their roots in poorly phrased comments at the dinner table. It's simply not the time to make remarks about weight or amounts eaten.

> Never bring anger to the table
> if you can help it.

And what's the best way to present the food at the table? Do you set the table or delegate it to another member of your household? If you have children, even the youngest members of the family can help with staging family meals. If you live alone, invite other people over to share the joys of your wonderful table. And let them help set the table or be part of the process. Even kids who have hours of homework can still take ten minutes to be part of an important family routine. They can learn to set the table by putting out placemats, napkins, and silverware for each member of the family. They can have fun by learning to decorate the table with their artwork or crafts, and they can fold napkins into fun shapes or designs. Their contribution may not be perfect but it will help them learn the importance of teamwork and the satisfaction of being part of the mealtime routine. And their help will save you a little time.

Clean-up is also an important part of the job. Clearing the table and sharing the dishwashing builds a sense of teamwork and commitment to help each other. Homework or the evening news can wait another few minutes.

Putting away leftovers may involve making individual portions of food that will be eaten for lunch the next day, or it might mean freezing extras for another day. Leaving leftovers out in plain sight may make it harder for some to avoid second helpings. And if you find that you are throwing away food that is not consumed, consider cooking less next time or donating food to those who don't have the means to eat as well as you do.

When you develop a plan of action to eat with intention and with others and to slow things down, try to start with the end in mind. In other words, start by envisioning your goal. For example, you might envision a video of you having a delicious, healthy, and relaxing meal at the end of the day. In today's hectic world it might be difficult for you to imagine a weekday evening when your favorite people, family, or close friends gather to share a beautiful and healthy meal together. How is that possible if you have a schedule that seems to include no time for preparing a healthy meal or to sit together, savoring the food and each other for an hour? Living a whole life takes time. It takes about thirty minutes for your brain to realize that you've eaten enough. It takes time for your stomach to register a level of satisfaction with a meal. And the spirit cannot be rushed at the sacred table.

> ## Delegate meal preparation
>
> Consider assigning meal preparation once a week to others who live in the house, a spouse or friend or a member of your community. If they don't have the necessary cooking skills, assign simple prep tasks such as peeling the vegetables or marinating the chicken. Everybody benefits.

Why wait until Thanksgiving to devote an entire day to enjoying food, family, and friends? Why wait to give thanks for the food we have available to us? Why not take some time each week or each day to feed your body and your soul at the same time and make meals part of the rhythm of your everyday life?

If you have neighbors or friends who are as busy as you, ask if they would like to alternate making dinner.

Maybe you'd like to begin by defining weeknight dinner. If you have neighbors or friends who are as busy as you, ask if they would like to alternate making dinner. This could mean hosting them for an evening meal this week and they would invite you next week. Some families have a "dinner club" more than once a week. My daughter and I used to alternate dinner once a week with a friend and her children when our husbands were away from home traveling on business. We found it eased our workload, provided much needed adult company, and gave the kids a chance to taste new foods.

This system allows you a night out for dinner without the expense of taking the family to a restaurant. It also provides companionship and the chance to try new dishes. If you schedule this for busy days, then it may help you avoid what often happens: a fast food meal or a take-out dinner that would be much higher in calories and more expensive than what you would eat at home or at a friend's house.

The habits that children develop at the family dinner table will influence their food choices when they are away from home in years to come. And although there is no single factor that leads to childhood obesity, research indicates that there is a connection between excess weight in childhood and how many meals are eaten with the family. Also, the more hours spent watching television, the greater the risk a child will gain excess weight. Alongside the sedentary aspect of television, snacking is often a part of the television habit. Overweight children who spend more TV time and less time at family meals are also more likely to stay overweight later in life.

I often see children in my practice who need to stop gaining weight and eat right. When I meet with the parents or the whole family, sometimes they come in with the idea that the child is the only one who needs to make changes in their eating and exercise habits. One young man who had been coming in with his sister and parents kept gaining weight instead of gradually losing weight. Every member of the family needed to eat better, exercise and lose weight. When he mentioned in one of our sessions that his dream was to go to one of the US military academies his eyes lit up and we began to discuss how the whole family could help to change their habits so that this young man could make his dream come true. Great things have happened since that family decided to make small steps toward a big goal. The strength training equipment was dusted off and a place was made in the basement for workouts. And they all started to walk on the local walking path on a regular basis. They are going to the local food pantry to find foods that can improve their family meals. This is an example of the small miracles that I witness every day. Even if this young man doesn't make it into a military academy he will have made an important change in his life that neither he nor his family will regret.

Build memories together. Take a walk before dinner or listen to your child practice the piano or harmonica after dinner. These are part of the precious family rituals that can be linked with family mealtime. One of my fondest memories at the dinner table was that of my daughter giving us a nightly ballet recital after dinner in the kitchen as my husband

and I sipped our coffee. My daughter did not become a professional dancer but the memory is a precious bond we all share.

You'll want to minimize distractions once you sit down to your meal. Turn off the television, cell phones, and pager. Stop text messaging. Devote yourself to the meal and the company. Imagine you are eating in a beautiful café or restaurant; play relaxing music in the background to change the hectic pace of the day during this sacred hour.

Table Time

Did you know that Americans spend less than one hour per day at the table, while the French spend two hours per day? Could eating leisurely be part of the "French Paradox," that is, their low incidence of heart disease despite their higher intake of fat?

We all tend to model eating habits after those we eat with, whether it's your spouse sitting across the table or your grandchildren watching you at Sunday brunch or your coworker in the lunchroom. I think it's especially difficult for women to find the portions that work for them when they are sitting across from their husbands who may be taller, more physically active, and need larger portions. And I've often seen a man gain weight during his wife's pregnancy, unconsciously increasing his food intake to keep pace with his wife's increased caloric needs.

Seven Secrets to Make Your Meals Sacred

- Express your thankfulness for each meal you eat.
- Make your meals a time-out from the hectic pace of life.
- Eat only in designated dining areas such as the kitchen, dining room, or backyard.
- Don't bring your worries or conflicts to the table.
- Laugh together at the table; share a joke or a funny story every night.
- Set the table to reflect the importance of the meal and those you are serving. Play music to change the mood. Light candles whenever you can at dinner. Enlist the help of others to set the table, serve the food, or clean up afterward.
- "Break bread together" whenever you can with those you love.

Celebrations, Splurges, and Sweets

M Y FATHER USED TO SAY, *"BONA FESTA, FESTA,"* or "When it's a feast, you feast." But in today's society feasting has become nearly a daily occurrence, rather than a special time to celebrate and enjoy the bounty of the season and treats that we seldom have. In my practice I often find that some of my clients not only have a sweet with lunch and dinner, but they also start the day with a sweetened cereal containing the same calories as a cookie or a muffin and nutritionally identical to a frosted cupcake. So by all means, feast when there's a reason, but don't make every day a feast day.

In the Recommended Daily Portion Guidelines (Appendix A) I've suggested portions of core foods and "your choice calories" that you can choose to round out your day's intake. You can use the extra calories for a larger portion of any of the food group portions, or you can choose a food that is outside the guidelines. The more calories you expend and need to eat, the easier it is to meet your intake of the core foods and use the additional calories to consume more core foods or a dessert, a special beverage, or other item of your choosing.

Unfortunately I often see individuals, both adults and children, who are consuming fewer whole healthy foods at the same time as they are consuming large amounts of sweets and processed foods. And it seems that the more sugar, fat, and salt they consume, the less appetite they have for fruits, vegetables, and whole grains. And the reverse is true; when you eat enough fruits, vegetables, and whole grains, your body may be less likely to constantly crave sweets. And although I have never seen a scientific study on this, perhaps if your mind, body, and spirit are properly nourished, that balance may have an impact on decreasing cravings for unhealthy foods. I have certainly seen this effect on individuals who I work with. The more healthy foods they include in their meals and snacks, the less they seem to crave addictive foods.

> When you eat enough fruits, vegetables, and whole grains, your body may be less likely to constantly crave sweets.

In our current food culture it is usually much easier to find a quick snack that is sweet, over-refined, and low in nutrients and fiber. It's not impossible, but it is more difficult, to walk into a store and find fruit or a genuine whole-grain snack. In fact many sweet snacks are labeled with health claims such as "low-fat" but fail to state on the label that they are high in added sugars. Many snack bars are really cookies in disguise. It's not that these foods can't be included in an otherwise healthy diet, but if we don't consider these foods as sweets, we may consume more sweets or desserts in the course of a day or a week than we realize. So if you would like to enjoy a dish of ice cream tonight after dinner, then you might consider snacking on some fruit or peanut butter on a whole-grain cracker rather than grabbing a candy bar at 4 PM.

Examples of Desserts in Disguise

- Sweetened yogurt
- Sweetened cereal or granola
- Snack bars
- Sweetened dried fruits
- Sweetened soda or iced tea
- Some flavored waters
- Some flavored coffee or tea drinks
- Commercial muffins and breakfast pastries
- Some dipping sauces

But you may wish to choose a healthier dessert, so consider including fruit as a dessert. It is a great way to satisfy your need for something sweet after lunch or dinner and still keep your caloric intake reasonable. If you do choose to have a sweet dessert such as chocolate, keep the portion small and savor the taste, letting it melt in your mouth for as long as possible. You may also want to serve fruit alongside a sweet dessert to give yourself and your guests a choice.

One new trend that I have seen in restaurants is the "mini-dessert." For a couple of dollars, you can get a miniature sample of a regular dessert such as carrot cake or chocolate mousse. After sampling this type of dessert, I bought attractive 2-ounce shot glasses and now use this technique when I have company for dinner. With this size serving, you have about 3 to 4 spoonfuls of a rich dessert but only a fraction of the calories. Even sharing a 600-Calorie piece of cake or other restaurant dessert provides far more calories than the "shot" of dessert.

Hospitality

Extending hospitality and welcoming others into our homes generally involves food no matter what our ethnic, cultural, or religious traditions. In Saint Benedict of Nursia's time hospitality included bed and board as well. "Let everyone that comes be received as Christ," the sixth-century abbot directed in the *Rule* for his monastery. In our society we still invite friends and family to come and stay with us, but more often hospitality means inviting others to lunch or dinner.

When entertaining we express our friendship, love, and caring through food. We express our own style of cooking, our own way of decorating the table, and perhaps the selection of music we play during the meal. Consideration for our guests can and should extend to serving healthy as well as delicious food.

When inviting guests to your home for a meal, be sure to ask if anyone has a food allergy, is vegetarian or vegan, or has

> When entertaining we express our friendship, love, and caring through food.

any particular medical nutritional needs that should be considered. During the summer I invited some friends for a backyard cookout. Although we have been friends for years and I knew that one of the guests has diabetes, I didn't realize that he had recently had extensive dental work. When Peter saw that fresh corn coming off the grill, he asked if I minded if he cut his off the cob. If I had known he couldn't chew well, I would have included more items on my menu to accommodate his needs. I also serve meals family-style or buffet-style when having friends and family for dinner. I usually print out the menu, listing each item for each course. This allows guests to make their own selections, choose their own portion size, and pace themselves by knowing what's coming next. If I do plate a meal to achieve a particular presentation, I always start by serving small portions and then provide second helpings for those who need or want them. Probably, for this reason, my friend Dennis always comments that when he dines at my table, he never feels that he has eaten too much and he feels quite satisfied.

I think that one of the dilemmas we face when trying to eat right is how to deal with food that is served to us by family and friends. Love and hospitality are so often expressed with food. One of the questions I am most frequently asked by clients is, "How can I eat right when my friends or family serve me rich foods that I am trying to avoid?"

Practice a response that works for you. Planning in advance will help you enjoy good food without overdoing it. And you can still be a grateful and gracious guest.

Polite Ways to Avoid Eating More Than You Need WHEN YOU'RE A GUEST

Delay: "No thanks. Maybe I'll try some later."

Decline: "The meal was so delicious;

I just don't have room for anything else."

Declare: "Everything looks so good,

but I've cut my portions and I'm satisfied with less now."

Defer on second helpings:

"Thanks, but I don't eat seconds anymore."

Hospitality involves the guest as well as the host. So if you have a dietary restriction, an allergy, or any other food intolerance, please let your host or hostess know. For example, if a person has celiac disease, careful preparation and handling of the food to avoid contamination with gluten is absolutely necessary. If you find yourself presented with foods that do not meet your medical needs, then eat only what is appropriate for you. As a guest, go to the table with an open heart as well as a flexible palate. Accept what you are served graciously and express your thanks.

Here is an example of an elegant but healthy meal that can be served for a crowd for a special occasion. It contains lean protein, nutrient-rich vegetables and fruits, healthy fats, and whole grains. Keep portions moderate to keep the calories moderate. Recipes are included for menu items in bold type.

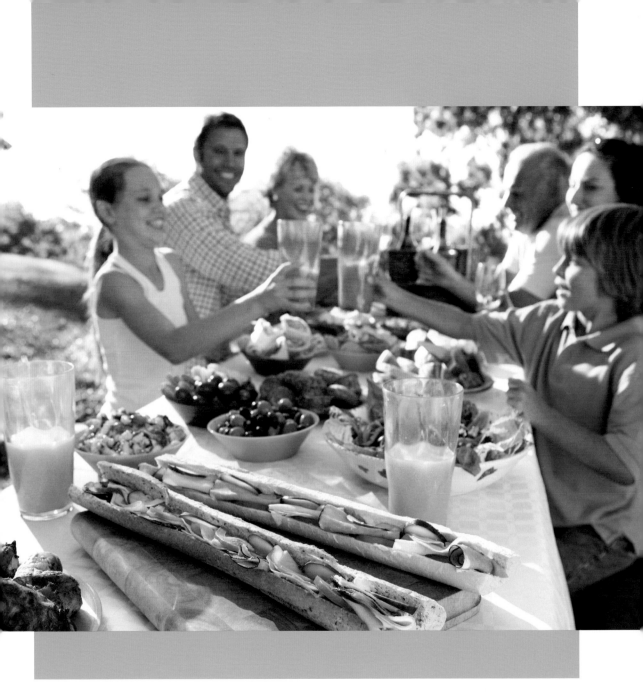

Don't wait for holidays
to share good food with family and friends.

Purchase the freshest
seasonal produce you can find.

Tomato Harvest Salad

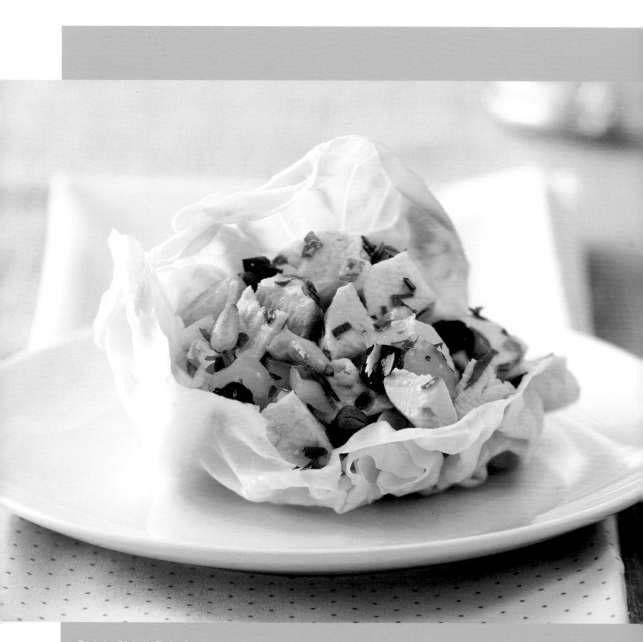

Quick Chick Salad

Thin Crust Pizza

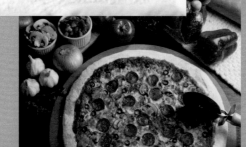

Personalize your
homemade pizza by offering
an array of vegetable toppings

Corny Southwestern Cornbread

Tomato and Fennel Bisque

Oven Roasted Vegetables

Classic
   Roasted Chicken

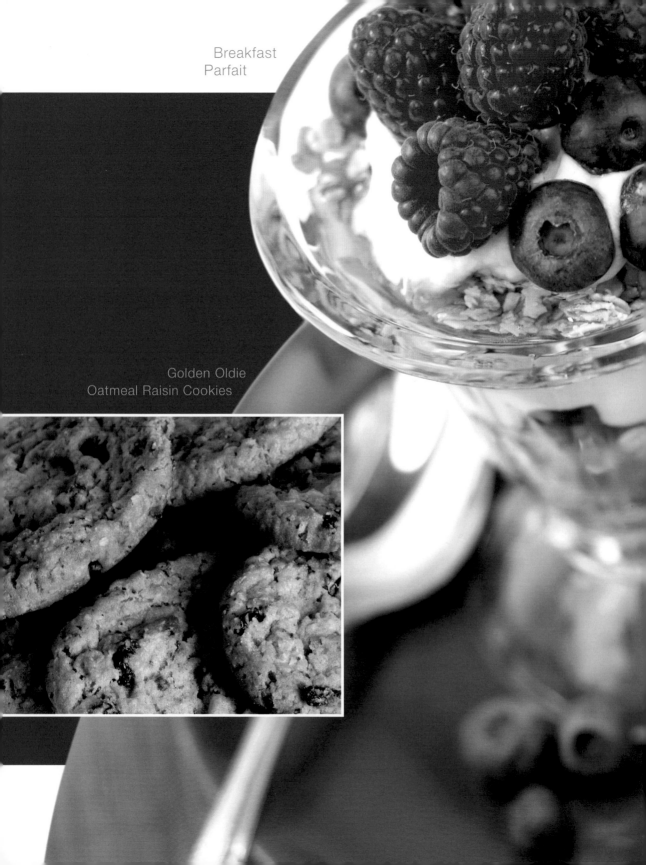

Breakfast
Parfait

Golden Oldie
Oatmeal Raisin Cookies

Celebration Dinner Menu

Shrimp with **Romesco Sauce**
Assorted Olives
Hummus with Vegetables and Whole-Grain Crackers

Five-Spice Pork Pot Roast
Gingered Winter Squash
Sesame Asparagus or **Green Beans and Shallots**

Whole Wheat Baguette and Olive Oil

Spiced Poached Fruit
Gingersnap Cookies

● ● ● ● ● ● ● ● ● ● ● ● ● ● ● ●

Hospitality Hints

- Ask your guests in advance if they have food allergies, medical diets, or particular food preferences that need to be considered.
- Let your guests know what the meal schedule will be.
- Include a variety of choices of vegetables, fruits, and whole grains along with special treats.
- Include dishes and menu items that are seasonal and appropriate to the event.
- Never encourage guests to overeat.
- Remember that a shared meal nourishes and honors the body, the mind, and the spirit.

Good Food Away from Home

I don't like to eat snails. I prefer fast food.
—Strange de Jim (1943–)

DO YOU GIVE UP WHEN YOU EAT OUT? Is it an excuse for abandoning your best-laid eating plans as well as your nutritional goals? Despite your eating right most of the time, dining out can add unplanned calories and sabotage your goals with less healthy foods and distorted portions. For example, you could be reducing your intake by 100 Calories a day. At a restaurant, though, you can easily consume an extra 700 Calories in one meal, cancelling out the daily reduction for the week. So let's look at developing a practical eating-out plan.

Eating meals away from home is a common necessity for those of us who work or go to school. Dining out with friends can be a wonderful pleasure. And take-out food can be the basis of a healthy meal when enhanced by a fresh food item at

Dining out with friends can be a wonderful pleasure. And take-out food can be the basis of a healthy meal when enhanced by a fresh food item at home.

home. Also, everyone loves having someone else set the table and do the dishes, as well as prepare and serve the meal. This can be a welcome break from the everyday meal routine. But if you often find yourself eating out in desperation because you haven't made plans for a meal at home, or you want to overindulge on rich foods, then you are headed for nutritional disaster.

If you eat more than two meals a week away from home, then you are having more than 10 percent of your meals away. If you eat one meal a day away from home, you are eating 33 percent of your meals away. And when you are traveling on business or on vacation, you are probably eating all of your meals out.

Yes, it's still possible to make good choices but it's definitely more challenging than eating at home or in a familiar restaurant. The more meals you eat out, the more carefully you need to plan. Learn to be conscious when ordering from a menu, helping yourself at a buffet or breakfast bar, or being a guest at someone's home. Making food decisions in advance rather than making impulsive or impromptu food choices can be a valuable discipline. Disciplining ourselves to eat right is a positive experience that can move us forward in our quest to include good food in our whole life. The routine of eating right every day does not have to be perceived as a negative behavior or as "boring." It is the type of discipline that over time establishes better habits.

Think You Can't Change?
CHANGE YOUR EXPECTATIONS

On her first visit to my office Geraldine told me that now that she was widowed and her kids were grown, she had been eating out nearly every meal for months. Dinner was often take-out or fast food. She had come to see me because she had just developed diabetes and her weight was at an all-time high. She was motivated to come in for advice since she didn't want to take medication if it wasn't truly necessary. She had been referred to me by another client, who warned me, "Good luck! She'll be tough to change!"

> My client had been "treating" herself by choosing to eat out every day but had turned her thinking around and now was "treating" her spirit with better foods and her body with greater care and respect.

But by my second visit with Geraldine, she had lost 4 pounds in four weeks and was preparing more of her meals at home. She told me jokingly that I had ruined fast food for her, now that she knew the facts about what she had been eating. Before, she had been "treating" herself by choosing to eat out every day but had turned her thinking around and now was "treating" her spirit with better foods and her body with greater care and respect. She had bought frozen vegetables and was microwaving them to enhance simple meals. When she did eat out she was ordering differently. She had even starting walking, and she was feeling more energy. During that month between our visits she had examined what she valued at this point in her life and realized that she wanted to stay healthy. She came in telling me about where she wanted her life to go in the next twenty years. By making the decision to control her weight and her diabetes, Geraldine now has a much better chance of reaching her lifestyle goals—something that she really hadn't expected!

Perhaps you have already started to plan lunches for work or school. If you're bringing lunch, then you have a good chance of eating a nourishing meal. Do you find yourself running out of fuel and looking for a candy bar to energize you? You may also need to bring snacks or stock your workplace with good food choices that are not perishable, or items like yogurt and cheese if you have access to a refrigerator.

If it's necessary to eat lunch in a restaurant or buy take-out, you can consult the Web to find menus that include the nutritional content of the food items offered in your favorite local or chain restaurants. Think of the online information as the equivalent of a food label for an item you might see in the grocery store. You may be choosing a salad for your lunch meal but you could compare the content of various salads and salad dressings to see what you are actually choosing. Maybe by making a simple switch you could save 100 Calories or 10 grams of fat without feeling deprived. Even comparing the portion size of menu items can make a difference in what you order. For example, what's the difference in the content of a cup of soup or a bowl of soup? The bowl could be 50 percent more or it could be double the portion.

Below is an example of the difference in what we can make at home and what we are served in a restaurant. I've listed two food items—one is my homemade Tomato and Fennel Bisque (see chapter 12 for the recipe) and the other version is a restaurant item. In this case the difference in nutrient content is dramatic; for example, the fat content is seven times greater in the restaurant version. And yet you may not have any idea when you're ordering that this kind of difference exists.

Tomato and Fennel Bisque
(Homemade)

Nutrition Facts

Serving Size (270g)
Servings Per Container

Amount Per Serving

Calories 110   Calories from Fat 35

	% Daily Value*
Total Fat 4g	**6%**
Saturated Fat 1g	**5%**
Trans Fat 0g	
Cholesterol 0mg	**0%**
Sodium 520mg	**22%**
Total Carbohydrate 16g	**5%**
Dietary Fiber 3g	**12%**
Sugars 9g	
Protein 5g	

Vitamin A 25%	•	Vitamin C 40%	
Calcium 6%	•	Iron 6%	

*Percent Daily Values are based on a 2,000 calorie diet. Your daily values may be higher or lower depending on your calorie needs:

		Calories:	2,000	2,500
Total Fat	Less than		65g	80g
Saturated Fat	Less than		20g	25g
Cholesterol	Less than		300mg	300mg
Sodium	Less than		2,400mg	2,400mg
Total Carbohydrate			300g	375g
Dietary Fiber			25g	30g

Calories per gram:
Fat 9 • Carbohydrate 4 • Protein 4

Tomato and Fennel Bisque
(Restaurant Item)

Nutrition Facts

Serving Size (294g)
Servings Per Container

Amount Per Serving

Calories 380   Calories from Fat 260

	% Daily Value*
Total Fat 29g	**45%**
Saturated Fat 13g	**65%**
Trans Fat 0g	
Cholesterol 65mg	**22%**
Sodium 1660mg	**69%**
Total Carbohydrate 25g	**8%**
Dietary Fiber 4g	**16%**
Sugars 11g	
Protein 6g	

Vitamin A 25%	•	Vitamin C 40%	
Calcium 6%	•	Iron 6%	

*Percent Daily Values are based on a 2,000 calorie diet. Your daily values may be higher or lower depending on your calorie needs:

		Calories:	2,000	2,500
Total Fat	Less than		65g	80g
Saturated Fat	Less than		20g	25g
Cholesterol	Less than		300mg	300mg
Sodium	Less than		2,400mg	2,400mg
Total Carbohydrate			300g	375g
Dietary Fiber			25g	30g

Calories per gram:
Fat 9 • Carbohydrate 4 • Protein 4

If fast food is your only option, then seek out at least one item for your meal that is a fruit or vegetable (no, I don't mean French fries . . .). Ask to have your sandwich without the heavy sauces and with extra lettuce and tomato. Avoid the trap of so-called special-value meals. There is no value in being served unhealthy food at a reduced price. Order water, low-fat milk, or unsweetened tea for your beverage. Skip the extra calories that are in the sodas and specialty waters. Share the entrée with a friend or take half home if the portion is more than you want.

The possibilities are endless
for eating healthier when away from home.

The possibilities are endless for eating healthier when away from home, but you must be a conscious eater and consider the options when choosing. That means shutting off "cruise control" on your journey to eat right. You may find it easier to decide in advance what you will order when you know you will be eating out. Don't think that you always need to order the Chicken Parmesan in your favorite Italian restaurant, even though you may have done so the past twenty times you were there. Decide in advance to order something **different and healthier** the next time and stick to your plan.

Beware of salty, fatty appetizers, since they can really increase your desire to eat. Let's face it—most of us don't need to have

Look for "Small Portion" Options on Menus

- Tasting portions
- Small Plates
- Samplers
- Half portions
- Contorni (Italian for side dishes)
- Tapas (Spanish for small snacks)
- Sharing portions

our appetites increased before we eat dinner. Instead consider what I call a first course. This starter item could be a clear soup or a crisp salad that is not laden with fat or cheese. The first course can make a significant contribution to the nutritional value and satisfaction of the meal. Whereas a fried appetizer, a Caesar salad, or any salty, fatty item can actually make you hungrier, a lighter item like a mixed garden salad with a low-fat dressing can make you feel satisfied sooner and eat less of the main course.

And try not to bring along your membership card to the Clean Plate Club when you eat out. The large portions served somehow trigger our brain to want to eat more. So splitting orders or asking for the take-home container before you start eating can be an important step to downsizing the message to your brain that you need to finish what was served.

Strategies for Eating Right
WHEN YOU'RE AWAY FROM HOME

- Research your menu choices in advance online or by phone.
- Don't be afraid to ask how a food is prepared before ordering in a restaurant.
- Bring a healthy dish with you to potluck suppers and gatherings with friends. If you know that rich food may be your only choice at a party, then bring a dish that you will be comfortable eating and that you will find satisfying.

- Take food with you when traveling by car, bus, train, or plane since your choices for good food will be limited, expensive, and often time-consuming.
- Don't give in when you eat out. Stick to your plan.

When you are trying to change habits, including how you eat when you're away from home, it's best to start with small changes. You might experiment with changing only one item on your main plate. For example, order a salad instead of the fries, or choose broiled fish instead of fried. Don't try to change your usual habits all at once. It can be helpful to try to make changes in the context of doing small experiments. Testing out different menu selections can help you gradually build the confidence to try more changes in the future. Remember, each new choice and each new habit will help you on your journey to making good food part of your whole life.

Eating Right for a Lifetime

Nothing would be more tiresome than eating and drinking if
God had not made them a pleasure as well as a necessity.
—Voltaire (1694–1778)

B Y THE TIME YOU FINISH READING THIS BOOK, you will probably have made some important changes in planning, preparing, and sharing good healthy food each day. The suggestions in each chapter have given you some ideas for making small but significant changes. But don't stop there! You may have tried some of my suggestions for getting organized or for changing your dinner routine. You may want to go back to those action plans to dig a little deeper to begin another layer of change. Or you may have already tried and accomplished most of the recommendations. Now is the time to assess what work still needs to be done. Some changes may have become automatic—for instance, lighting a candle every night at the dinner table or using placemats at the counter for breakfast, to create a meaningful space and time.

Other issues may require your focus and commitment for some time to come. The journey to a whole life is never really over. We must continue to try to eat good food even as our needs change with age. We may need to redefine living well as we get older. And we should get to know our mind, body, and soul even better each day of our lives.

> Now is the time to assess
> what work still needs to be done.

And life sometimes imposes changes on us that we hadn't planned for, such as a change in the size of your family or the members of your household. Some individuals may have to deal with their grown children moving back into the family home along with their children if they lose their jobs. Newlyweds will have to make changes if children come along, and those in middle age may need to adjust as the nest empties or after the loss of a spouse or parent. I recall the adjustments in my cooking for my husband after we were married. As the oldest daughter of a large family, I was used to cooking very large meals, especially for my brothers who were athletes and were ravenous by dinnertime.

I started to downsize soon after my wedding by cutting my favorite recipes in half and saving the rest for another meal. I had to continue to decrease the amount I was cooking until it was just right for two. If I had continued to cook the amount of food and the type of food that I cooked for my brothers when they were playing football or hockey, I would have gained weight and been much less healthy. And now as my husband and I get older, we seem to need less each year. We continue to decrease the amount of food we buy and the amount we prepare.

As a practicing Registered Dietitian and nutritionist I try to learn more each day in order to give the best information and advice I can to my clients. At the same time I realize that making choices to eat right and learning new information and skills about healthy lifestyles is a daily challenge for my clients as well for the rest of us.

Don't think you have to be perfect to eat right. I prefer striving for excellence over "perfection." Would you ever criticize someone who tried hard to be excellent at his or her work or an exceptional parent? No. Being human, we may never achieve perfection in eating right, but we can make the best choices possible each day if we make it a priority. And if you make a poor choice,

> Don't think you have to be perfect to eat right. I prefer striving for excellence over "perfection."

and we all do, begin again. So keep the title of this book in mind—*Good Food for Life*—and make the best plans you can for eating right each day for the rest of your life.

As you understand by now, this book is not a "diet" book. It does not offer a day-to-day plan that dictates exactly what you should eat. It is a guidebook for applying the principles of eating right. I hope you will use it as a road map on your journey to consuming good food for life. Learning to eat right is a lot like learning a new language. Initially you learn the nouns, verbs, adjectives, and a few expressions, but you still have to consciously translate from your native language into the new one. As you practice more or are immersed in the culture on a trip to the foreign country, you learn to put sentences together and learn common phrases by heart. Fluency comes when you no longer need to translate before you speak. You speak intuitively in the new language, that is, you don't need to stop and think in your native language before speaking. Eating well is like learning that new language. And it's a language in which I hope you develop great fluency!

You may not need this book every day, but I hope that you reread it, chapter by chapter, whenever your circumstances change. You may also want to use it to help you transition your meals from one season to another using available produce. And I hope it helps you move toward good food for your own life every day. Keep planning, preparing, and sharing!

Sample Menus and Recipes

To eat is a necessity; to eat intelligently is an art.
—François de La Rochefoucald (1613–1680)

Meal and Snack Inspirations

YOU'LL FIND SAMPLE MENUS FOR EACH SEASON OF THE YEAR. The menu selections for each season are representative of the types of food that are available during that time of year. Of course many items such as green beans or strawberries are picked at the height of the season and frozen so they are available year round.

The sample menus are just that—samples. They are designed to give you examples of how you can plan meals that are seasonally appropriate and incorporate more fruits, vegetables, and whole grains into your everyday meals. The menus include ideas for breakfasts, lunches, dinners, and snacks and also suggestions for how you might choose to use your extra food choices. You may choose to focus just on planning your lunches at first. Or you could plan to try three family dinners.

I have also given an example of how a menu could be served at the 1600- and 2200-Calorie levels. You can log on to www.3DYourWholeLife.com to find more menus for specific calorie levels. Although the 1600-Calorie menus average 1600 Calories per day, in real life you may eat 1400 or 1500 Calories some days and other days you might eat 1700 or 1800 Calories. Measurements in a home kitchen are generally done with household measuring utensils or by eye. And the nutrient content of fresh foods can vary from season to season, depending on the level of ripeness or the method of preparation. So even if you use a computer or a food composition book, you may not always get exactly the nutrient content you think you're consuming. Aim for a daily routine of seeking out good food, eating when you're hungry, and stopping when you're satisfied. Even if you're not focused on managing your weight, just planning on having enough fruit, vegetables, and whole grains will take time and effort and reap rewards as well!

Spring Menu

Sunday

breakfast	lunch	dinner	snack	your choice
Asparagus on Toast **Mock Hollandaise Sauce** Fresh Strawberries	Asian Vegetable Patties Pineapple Chunks Mesclun Salad Ginger Cookies	Grilled Steak **Baked Barley Mushroom Risotto** Beets Wax Beans	Honeydew Melon Vanilla Nonfat Greek Yogurt	**Pumpkin Pie Pudding**

Monday

breakfast	lunch	dinner	snack	your choice
Egg Sandwich on English Muffin Roasted Red Pepper	Nicoise Salad w/oil & vinegar: Tuna Green Beans Potato Hard-boiled Egg Whole Wheat Roll & Olive Oil	**Classic Roasted Chicken** Swiss Chard **Stuffed Roasted Onions** Crusty Whole Grain Roll or Bread Strawberry Rhubarb Fruit Crisp	Low Fat Fudgsicle Green Grapes	Butter or Olive Oil

Tuesday

breakfast	lunch	dinner	snack	your choice
Grapefruit Half Whole Grain Toast Almond Butter	Cooked Shrimp Tabouleh Salad Kiwi	Pork Tenderloins with Dry Rub Mustard **Sweet and Sour Red Cabbage** **Green Beans and Shallots** Rye Bread	Uncle Sam's cereal Nonfat milk Sliced Strawberries	Nutella Spread Banana

Wednesday

breakfast	lunch	dinner	snack	your choice
Breakfast Parfait Apple	Cuban Sandwich: Pulled Pork Pickles or Sliced Cucumbers Shredded Green Cabbage Whole Wheat Roll	**Bolognese Sauce** Wide Noodles Arugula Salad Parmesan Cheese Fresh Fruit Cup **Cannoli Cream**	Banana Finn Crisp Crackers	Strawberries dipped in Dark Melted Chocolate

Thursday				
breakfast	lunch	dinner	snack	your choice
Weetabix Banana Sliced Almonds Nonfat Milk	Turkey Roll-up Asparagus Spears Mandarin Oranges	Beef Stew **Basic Green Salad** Whole Wheat Ciabatta Bread	Sugar Snap Peas or Pea Pods Red Pepper Strips Red Pepper Hummus	Rioja Wine

Friday				
breakfast	lunch	dinner	snack	your choice
Egg White & Vegetable Omelet Toasted Sprouted Bread Olive Oil Pineapple Slices	**Cheesy Waldorf Salad** Breadstick	**Parchment Pesce** Quinoa Matchstick Vegetables Coffee Ice Cream	Air-popped Corn	Canned Pear Half with Chocolate Syrup

Saturday				
breakfast	lunch	dinner	snack	your choice
Wheatena or Multigrain Hot Cereal Tangelo or Clementine Nonfat Milk	Salmon Salad Sprouted Flax Bread Grape Tomatoes **Asian Slaw** Fresh Fruit	**Ancho Chili Chicken Breast** Spring Greens Salad Light Corn Chips Shredded Cheese Salsa	VitaTop Muffin	Mexican Beer

Note: You'll find recipes in this book for menu items listed in bold.

Summer Menu

Sunday

breakfast	lunch	dinner	snack	your choice
Cheerios Fresh Strawberries Nonfat Milk	Soy Burger Whole Grain Pita Red Onion Avocado wedges Salsa & Lettuce	**Tapenade Tuna** Sliced Fresh Tomato Corn on the Cob Basic Green Salad **Cannoli Cream** w/ Fresh Berries	Cantaloupe Prosciutto Slice	Lemonade Butter on Corn

Monday

breakfast	lunch	dinner	snack	your choice
Fresh Cantaloupe Low-fat Cottage Cheese Cinnamon Toasted Oat Bread	Seafood Salad on Greens **Sesame Asparagus** Fresh pineapple Gingersnaps	Grilled Chicken w/ **Gremolata** Eggplant Ratatouille Spinach Salad	Nectarine Mini Shredded Wheat Nonfat milk	Olive Oil Sourdough Bread

Tuesday

breakfast	lunch	dinner	snack	your choice
Summer Fruit Smoothie Corn Muffin	Manhattan Clam Chowder Garden Salad Greek Yogurt	Lean Burgers Green Beans Bulgur Tabouleh **Peach, Blueberry, and Lime Compote**	Low-fat Cheddar Triscuits	Pomegranate Juice Nuts

Wednesday

breakfast	lunch	dinner	snack	your choice
Fresh Fruit Cup English Muffin Peanut Butter	Smoked Salmon Kavli 5-Grain Crackers Sliced Cucumbers & Dill Bing Cherries	Grilled Shrimp Pasta with Pesto **Roasted Summer Vegetables** Sliced Tomatoes Mozzarella (Part Skim) Cheese	Fresh Apricot Maple Corn Muffin	Watermelon

Thursday

breakfast	**lunch**	**dinner**	**snack**	**your choice**
Vegetable Frittata Wedge Onion Bialy Papaya Slices	Roast Beef Wrap Horseradish Mayo **Dijon Potato Salad** Watermelon	Chunky Chicken Chili Corn Tortillas **Tomato Harvest Salad** Pluot or Fresh Apricots	Raw Vegetables Whole Wheat Pita Chips Garlic Hummus	Corn Muffin

Friday

breakfast	**lunch**	**dinner**	**snack**	**your choice**
Whole Grain Waffle Blackberries Light Vanilla Yogurt	**Quick Chick Salad** Fresh Greens Fresh Grapes Crepe or Oat Bran Wrap **Golden Oldie Oatmeal Raisin Cookie**	Spinach Lasagna Romaine Lettuce Yogurt Caesar Dressing Whole Wheat Baguette Olive Oil	Cottage Cheese Fresh Peach	Chianti

Saturday

breakfast	**lunch**	**dinner**	**snack**	**your choice**
Egg White Turkey Sausage Sandwich (take-out breakfast) Fresh Fruit from Home	**Shrimp, Cannellini & Tomatoes** Fresh Basil Olive Oil Crisp Leaf Lettuce Whole Grain Crackers	Cajun Turkey on the Grill Grilled Pineapple Slice Grilled Zucchini Spears Red Onion Slice Whole Wheat Buns	Watermelon **Two by Two Spiced Nuts**	Fruit Crisp

Fall Menu

Sunday

breakfast	lunch	dinner	snack	your choice
Whole Grain French Toast Frozen Berries Maple Syrup	**Anadama Batter Bread** Sliced Chicken Breast Marinated Cauliflower	Pork Loin Dried Fruit Stuffing Sauce/Gravy Applesauce Mashed Butternut Squash	**Nuts About Red Pepper Dip** Vegetable Spears	**Golden Oldie Oatmeal Raisin Cookie**

Monday

breakfast	lunch	dinner	snack	your choice
Low-fat Cottage Cheese Fruit Toasted Slivered Almonds Whole Grain Toast	Lentil Soup Akmak Crackers Spinach Salad Hard-boiled Egg Banana	**Triple Bean and Turkey Stew** Dark Green Salad & Italian Dressing Whole Wheat Roll Olive Oil Vanilla Ice Cream	Greek Yogurt Crushed Pineapple	Shortbread Cookie

Tuesday

breakfast	lunch	dinner	snack	your choice
Whole Wheat English Muffin Scrambled Eggs Sliced Tomato	**Smothered Soy Burger** Rye Bread **Lemon-marinated Vegetables** Dried Plums	Baked Haddock or Cod **Green Rice** **Orange Glazed Carrots** Fresh Fig	Macintosh Apple Gingersnaps	Asiago Cheese

Wednesday

breakfast	lunch	dinner	snack	your choice
Raisin Bran Muffins Fruit Cup	**Heavenly Turkey Sandwich** Ezekiel Bread Carrot Salad Fuji Apple	Frittata or Omelet Escarole Salad Manchego Cheese Pear	Dates Pistachios	Hot Cocoa

Thursday

breakfast	lunch	dinner	snack	your choice

Hot Multigrain Cereal
Dried Cranberries or
  Cherries
Low-fat Soymilk Milk
	Hummus
	Roasted Red
	  Peppers
	5 Grain Kavli Crackers
	Babybel Light
	  Cheese
	Dried Apricots
		London Broil
		Baked Potato
		  Wedges
		French Green Beans
		Shades of Red Salad
			Celery
			Peanut Butter
			Popcorn
				Italian Ice or Sorbet

Friday

breakfast	lunch	dinner	snack	your choice

Poached egg
Whole Wheat Toast
Nonfat Milk
Orange Juice
	**Red Chili Con
	  Carne**
	Chopped Red
	  Onions
	Chopped Plum
	  Tomatoes
	Shredded Low-fat
	  Cheese
	**Corny Southwestern
	  Cornbread**
		Curried Scallops or
		  Shrimp
		Angel hair pasta
		Broccoli
		Vegetable Soup
			Almond Butter
			Kavli Crackers
			Clementine
				**Maple-baked
				  Apples**

Saturday

breakfast	lunch	dinner	snack	your choice

Breakfast Burrito
Tangerine
	Leftover London
	  Broil Slices
	**Whole Grain &
	  Bean Salad**
	Yogurt & Crushed
	  Pineapple
		**Tomato and Fennel
		  Bisque**
		Grilled Chicken Thighs
		Broccoli
		Brown Basmati Rice
			Soy Joy Bar	Almond Biscotti

Winter Menu

Sunday

breakfast	lunch	dinner	snack	your choice
Make-ahead Oatmeal Grapefruit or Pummelo Sections Nonfat Milk	Homemade **Thin Crust Pizza** Broccoli Slaw Grapes	**Classic Roasted Chicken Roasted Roots** Fresh Asparagus **Fruit Crisp**	Greek Yogurt Tangelo	Popcorn Fresh Cranberry Sauce

Monday

breakfast	lunch	dinner	snack	your choice
Blueberry Smoothie Ezekiel Toast Peanut Butter	Turkey Roll-up on Whole Grain Wrap Avocado Sliced Cucumber Shredded Lettuce or Romaine Canned Pineapple	**Wild Mushroom Sauté with Whole-grain Pasta** Fresh Broccolini or Frozen Broccoli Parmesan Cheese Poached or Canned Pear	Low-fat Swiss Cheese Kavli Crackers Carrot and Pepper Sticks	Red Wine Pine Nuts

Tuesday

breakfast	lunch	dinner	snack	your choice
100% Shredded Wheat Banana Slices Nonfat Milk	**Whole-grain Grilled Cheese Sandwich** Minestrone Soup Chocolate Pudding	Pan-Grilled Steak Slices Roasted Brussels Sprouts Baked Sweet Potato Wedges **Marinated Cauliflower** Salad	All-Fruit Preserves Peanut Butter Whole Grain Wasa Crackers Fresh Fruit Cup	Vanilla Ice Cream Frozen Raspberries

Wednesday

breakfast	lunch	dinner	snack	your choice
Homemade or Starbuck's Oatmeal Frozen Berries Nonfat Milk	**Steak, Tomatoes & Artichoke Hearts** Golden Delicious Apple Baked Whole Wheat Pita Chips	**Savory Baked Tilapia** Lundberg Brown Rice Chopped Cooked Frozen Spinach **Pumpkin Pie Pudding**	Vegetable or Minestrone Soup Gingersnaps Orange Sections	Banana & Peanut Butter

Thursday				
breakfast	lunch	dinner	snack	your choice
Whole Grain Cereal Flakes Dried Strawberries Nonfat Milk	Tuna Sandwich on Rye Raw Vegetable Tidbits Fruit Salad	**Minted Pea Soup** **Hazelnut Turkey Burgers** Whole Wheat Burger Buns **Maple-baked Apples**	Low-fat Feta Cheese Chunks Olives Grape Tomatoes	Dark Chocolate Avocado Slices

Friday				
breakfast	lunch	dinner	snack	your choice
Vegetable Omelet **Wholesome "Hearty" Muffin** Melon Chunks	**Shrimp, Cannellini & Tomatoes** Raw Vegetable Tidbits Breadstick or Whole Grain Bread Fresh Clementine	**Portuguese Fish Stew** **Basic Green Salad** Whole Grain Bruschetta Low-fat Vanilla Ice Cream Mango Chunks	Dried Apricots Pistachios Hot Chocolate	Biscotti White Wine

Saturday				
breakfast	lunch	dinner	snack	your choice
Buckwheat or Whole Grain Waffles Frozen Berry Sauce Hot Chocolate	**Huevos a la Flamenca** Whole Wheat Baguette Slices Olive Oil	Chicken Sausage Fajitas Oat Bran Tortillas Low-fat Taco Cheese Grilled Peppers & Onions Jicama & Orange Salad Salsa & Avocado Garnish	Celery Stalks Lemon Hummus Tangerine	Mexican Beer or Cider Maple Syrup

Sample Recipes

Recipes in this collection are representative of various types of good food that can be part of your everyday meals and snacks. Recipe examples are drawn from different geographic regions, ethnic cuisines, seasons of the year, various cooking abilities, complexity of preparation, and cost. Some of them are my personal favorites and many were given to me by my clients or served to me by friends.

You'll find general portion sizes listed with the number of servings for each of the food groups and a nutrition facts label that makes it easy to see at a glance what the food item provides in a recipe serving.

Recipes included in this book are highlighted in bold on the sample menus. I've also included some ideas for food combinations that are classic, simple, and delicious. And in the Resources section I've given you my recommendations for additional recipe sources from books, magazines, and websites.

I hope you enjoy these delicious good foods as you plan your menus, prepare your meals, and share them with those you love!

Whole-Grain Favorites

- Barbara's Shredded Wheat (the only ingredient is organic whole grain)
- Uncle Sam's cereal
- Weetabix cereal
- Pinhead Scottish or Irish oatmeal (steel cut) or Old-Fashioned Rolled Oats
- Plain air-popped or microwaved regular popcorn
- Whole-grain crackers—Ryvita, Kavli, Wasa, Akmak, Finn Crisp
- Whole-grain sides—wheat berries, quinoa, whole-wheat bulgur or couscous, barley, Lundberg whole-grain rice
- Sprouted whole-grain breads and rolls—Ezekiel bread, Alvarado Street Bakery bread, Trader Joe's sprouted breads
- Barilla Plus pasta

Good Food for Life Recipes

Alphabetical Listing of Recipes

Blueberry Smoothie

Smoothies can be a great breakfast when you're in a rush. Measure the ingredients the night before and have the blender ready on the kitchen counter so that you'll have no reason to skip breakfast.

Mix all ingredients in a blender with 2 ice cubes until smooth.

¾ cup fresh or frozen
   unsweetened blueberries
¾ cup nonfat milk or original
   soy milk or light soy milk
2 tablespoons unsweetened
   soy protein powder or
   instant nonfat milk powder
¼ teaspoon lemon extract
¼ teaspoon vanilla extract
⅛ teaspoon cinnamon

Makes 1 serving.
Each serving counts as
1 fruit, 2 lean proteins,
and 1 high-calcium food.

Nutrition Facts

Calories 200	Calories from Fat 15

	% Daily Value*
Total Fat 1.5g	**2%**
Saturated Fat 0g	**0%**
Trans Fat 0g	
Cholesterol 5mg	**2%**
Sodium 100mg	**4%**
Total Carbohydrate 26g	**9%**
Dietary Fiber 3g	**12%**
Sugars 20g	
Protein 22g	

Vitamin A 20%	•	Vitamin C 20%	
Calcium 40%	•	Iron 2%	

*Percent Daily Values are based on a 2,000 calorie diet. Your daily values may be higher or lower depending on your calorie needs:

		Calories: 2,000	2,500
Total Fat	Less than	65g	80g
Saturated Fat	Less than	20g	25g
Cholesterol	Less than	300mg	300mg
Sodium	Less than	2,400mg	2,400mg
Total Carbohydrate		300g	375g
Dietary Fiber		25g	30g

Calories per gram:
Fat 9 • Carbohydrate 4 • Protein 4

Breakfast Burrito

• •

1 egg (or ¼ cup egg substitute)
¼ cup pre-cooked broccoli
   or asparagus
1 slice low-fat cheese
1 oat bran or whole-wheat
   tortilla (7–8 inch)
1 tablespoon pico de gallo
   (or fresh tomato salsa)

Makes 1 serving.
Each serving counts as 2 lean proteins, 2 starches, and 1 vegetable.

This doesn't take much more time than pulling into a fast food take-out window. You can make it with liquid egg substitute so you don't even have to crack an egg. And you can use a wide variety of low-fat cheeses and vegetables to vary this quick breakfast.

Scramble the egg. Place on the tortilla. Top with vegetable, cheese, and pico de gallo. Roll up and wrap in parchment paper. Cut in half right through the paper and enjoy.

Nutrition Facts

Calories 270	Calories from Fat 90

	% Daily Value*
Total Fat 10g	15%
Saturated Fat 3g	15%
Trans Fat 0g	
Cholesterol 215mg	72%
Sodium 640mg	27%
Total Carbohydrate 30g	10%
Dietary Fiber 3g	12%
Sugars 4g	
Protein 17g	

Vitamin A 15%	•	Vitamin C 30%	
Calcium 25%	•	Iron 15%	

*Percent Daily Values are based on a 2,000 calorie diet. Your daily values may be higher or lower depending on your calorie needs:

		Calories:	2,000	2,500
Total Fat	Less than		65g	80g
Saturated Fat	Less than		20g	25g
Cholesterol	Less than		300mg	300mg
Sodium	Less than		2,400mg	2,400mg
Total Carbohydrate			300g	375g
Dietary Fiber			25g	30g

Calories per gram:
Fat 9 • Carbohydrate 4 • Protein 4

Breakfast Parfait

● ● ● ● ● ● ● ● ● ● ● ● ● ● ● ● ● ● ●

A dish this simple really doesn't need a specific recipe since it's made of simple components that can be endlessly varied depending on the season and on what you have on hand.

Use a parfait glass, a goblet, a custard cup, or other glass container that will show off the layers of this parfait.

Start the layering by placing ¼ cup yogurt, then ¼ cup fruit. Add half the granola and then repeat the layers. Garnish with citrus zest for more color and flavor.

These can be made the night before for a quick breakfast at home, or you can take it with you to eat at work. The sugars on the nutrition label are from the yogurt and the fruit. There are no added sugars.

½–¾ cup plain nonfat Greek yogurt
½–¾ cup fresh or frozen berries or other seasonal fruit
¼ cup light granola or grape nuts
Lemon or lime zest
(optional garnish)

Makes 1 serving.
Each serving counts as 1 whole grain, 1 fruit, 1 lean protein, and 1 high-calcium food (but with fewer calories than expected because of the low-calorie and high-nutrient content of the Greek yogurt).

Nutrition Facts

Calories 190   Calories from Fat 15

	% Daily Value*
Total Fat 1.5g	**2%**
Saturated Fat 0g	**0%**
Trans Fat 0g	
Cholesterol 0mg	**0%**
Sodium 50mg	**2%**
Total Carbohydrate 31g	**10%**
Dietary Fiber 4g	**16%**
Sugars 8g	
Protein 15g	

Vitamin A 0%   •   Vitamin C 110%
Calcium 15%   •   Iron 8%

*Percent Daily Values are based on a 2,000 calorie diet. Your daily values may be higher or lower depending on your calorie needs:

	Calories:	2,000	2,500
Total Fat	Less than	65g	80g
Saturated Fat	Less than	20g	25g
Cholesterol	Less than	300mg	300mg
Sodium	Less than	2,400mg	2,400mg
Total Carbohydrate		300g	375g
Dietary Fiber		25g	30g

Calories per gram:
Fat 9 • Carbohydrate 4 • Protein 4

Make-ahead Oatmeal

2½ **cups old-fashioned oats
(not quick oats)**

⅓ **cup firmly packed brown sugar**

⅓ **cup dried cranberries or
chopped dried apricots**

⅓ **cup chopped toasted
walnuts or pecans**

1 **teaspoon cinnamon**

1 **teaspoon fresh ground nutmeg**

½ **teaspoon salt (optional)**

3 **cups nonfat milk**

1 **whole large egg and 3 egg
whites, lightly beaten, or**

1 **cup egg substitute**

2 **teaspoons vanilla extract**

**Makes 10 servings.
Each serving counts as 1 whole
grain, 1 fat, and 1 protein.**

There's no excuse to skip a hot breakfast with this make-ahead version of oatmeal. It's also great if you're having a crowd for breakfast. One serving made with brown sugar has 7 grams of added sugar, so if you want to omit this from the recipe you will reduce the Calories to 160 instead of 190, and the carb content will be 22 grams instead of 29 grams.

Preheat oven to 350 degrees. Spray a 2-quart glass or ceramic baking dish with cooking spray. Toss the dry ingredients in a large bowl to mix. In a 1-quart glass measuring cup or bowl, blend the liquid ingredients together and add to the dry ingredients, mixing well. Pour the mixture into the prepared baking dish. Bake for approximately 1 hour (check at 45 minutes since oven temperatures can vary widely). When the center is set and firm it's done. Cool for 5 minutes and serve immediately, or cover tightly and store leftovers in the refrigerator for up to five days.

Individual servings of the baked oatmeal can be reheated in the microwave, adding additional water if necessary to get the consistency you like.

Nutrition Facts		
Calories 190 Calories from Fat 40		
		% Daily Value*
Total Fat 4.5g		**7%**
Saturated Fat 0g		**0%**
Trans Fat 0g		
Cholesterol 20mg		**7%**
Sodium 65mg		**3%**
Total Carbohydrate 29g		**10%**
Dietary Fiber 3g		**12%**
Sugars 14g		
Protein 9g		
Vitamin A 4%	• Vitamin C 0%	
Calcium 10%	• Iron 6%	

*Percent Daily Values are based on a 2,000 calorie diet. Your daily values may be higher or lower depending on your calorie needs:

	Calories:	2,000	2,500
Total Fat	Less than	65g	80g
Saturated Fat	Less than	20g	25g
Cholesterol	Less than	300mg	300mg
Sodium	Less than	2,400mg	2,400mg
Total Carbohydrate		300g	375g
Dietary Fiber		25g	30g

Calories per gram:
Fat 9 • Carbohydrate 4 • Protein 4

Wholesome "Hearty" Muffins

· · · · · · · · · · · · · · · · · ·

These muffins get their moistness from oat bran and applesauce. They are so easy to make that you can delegate your children to measure and mix them. They freeze well and reheat in the microwave in less than 30 seconds on a cold morning for a heart-healthy breakfast or snack. They have less than half the calories of store-bought muffins and cost much less to make.

⅓ cup packed light brown sugar
1½ cups oat bran
1 cup unbleached white flour
½ cup whole-wheat flour
1½ teaspoon baking soda
1½ teaspoon baking powder
½ teaspoon salt
4 egg whites (or 2 whole large eggs)
1 cup unsweetened applesauce
¼ cup canola, grape seed, or light olive oil
½ cup frozen blueberries or golden raisins

Spray 12 muffin cups with non-stick spray.
Preheat oven to 400 degrees.
Place dry ingredients into a bowl or 2-quart glass measuring cup.

Add eggs, applesauce, and oil to dry ingredients and mix just until ingredients are combined (do not over-beat).
Pour or spoon batter into the muffin tin.
Bake approximately 15 minutes or until lightly browned.

Makes 12 muffins.
Each muffin counts as
1 whole grain, 1 starch,
½ protein, and 1 fat.

Nutrition Facts		
Calories 170	Calories from Fat 50	
		% Daily Value*
Total Fat 6g		9%
Saturated Fat 0.5g		3%
Trans Fat 0g		
Cholesterol 0mg		0%
Sodium 340mg		14%
Total Carbohydrate 30g		10%
Dietary Fiber 3g		12%
Sugars 8g		
Protein 6g		
Vitamin A 0%	• Vitamin C 0%	
Calcium 2%	• Iron 8%	

*Percent Daily Values are based on a 2,000 calorie diet. Your daily values may be higher or lower depending on your calorie needs:

		Calories:	2,000	2,500
Total Fat	Less than		65g	80g
Saturated Fat	Less than		20g	25g
Cholesterol	Less than		300mg	300mg
Sodium	Less than		2,400mg	2,400mg
Total Carbohydrate			300g	375g
Dietary Fiber			25g	30g

Calories per gram:
Fat 9 • Carbohydrate 4 • Protein 4

Ancho Chili Chicken Breast

1 shallot, finely chopped
1 garlic clove, finely chopped
2 tablespoons finely chopped
  fresh chives or
  2 teaspoons dried chives
3 tablespoons chopped fresh cilantro
  or parsley
1 tablespoon ancho chili powder
1 teaspoon ground cumin
3 tablespoons olive oil
  Juice of 1 lime
  Salt and pepper to taste (optional)
2 pounds boneless, skinless
  chicken breasts
1 pineapple, peeled, cored,
  and sliced into 8 slices
  Fresh lime wedges for garnish
  Fresh cilantro leaves for garnish

Makes 8 servings.
Each serving counts as 4 proteins
and 1 fruit.

Ancho chili powder gives this chicken a distinctive taste of chili peppers but it's not fiery hot. You can always substitute any chili powder you have on hand. Grilling fruit and serving with meat can add nutrition and color, and it's so easy to do while the grill is already hot.

Place the first 9 ingredients into a small glass measuring pitcher and whisk together until the herbs and spices are incorporated into the marinade.

Place the chicken breasts in a pie pan or a shallow marinating container. Pour the ancho chili marinade over the chicken. Turn the breasts over once to coat thoroughly. Cover and place in the refrigerator overnight or at least 4 hours. Before cooking, drain the marinade and let the chicken breasts come to room temperature to maximize tenderness.

Heat a gas grill for 10 minutes using a medium flame. Oil the grill grates using tongs and a paper towel moistened with 1 tablespoon of peanut or canola oil. Place the chicken breasts over the flame for 3–4 minutes per side to brown. Move them to a part of the grill that does not have a flame and cover the grill. Cook for another 8–12 minutes, depending on the thickness of the meat. Check to make sure the internal temperature reaches 165 degrees. Remove chicken from the grill and cover with foil for another 5–10 minutes.

In the meantime, place the pineapple slices on the grill and cook for 3–4 minutes per side.

Slice the chicken breasts as you would a roast or steak. Arrange on a platter with the grilled pineapple and fresh cilantro.

Nutrition Facts

Calories 170	Calories from Fat 20	
		% Daily Value*
Total Fat 2g		3%
Saturated Fat 0g		0%
Trans Fat 0g		
Cholesterol 65mg		22%
Sodium 75mg		3%
Total Carbohydrate 11g		4%
Dietary Fiber 1g		4%
Sugars 8g		
Protein 27g		
Vitamin A 2%	•	Vitamin C 70%
Calcium 2%	•	Iron 6%

*Percent Daily Values are based on a 2,000 calorie diet. Your daily values may be higher or lower depending on your calorie needs:

		Calories:	2,000	2,500
Total Fat	Less than		65g	80g
Saturated Fat	Less than		20g	25g
Cholesterol	Less than		300mg	300mg
Sodium	Less than		2,400mg	2,400mg
Total Carbohydrate			300g	375g
Dietary Fiber			25g	30g

Calories per gram:
Fat 9 • Carbohydrate 4 • Protein 4

Bolognese Sauce

On one of my trips to Italy I had Pasta Bolognese in a little trattoria near the Church of St. Dominic in Bologna. It was simple and elegant, rich and meaty, served with wide ribbon-shaped pasta called papardelle. You can also serve it with whole-wheat fettuccini or with spaghetti such as Barilla Plus, which contains extra protein, fiber, and other nutrients.

3   tablespoons extra virgin olive oil
1   large onion
1   large carrot
3   stalks of celery, leaves included
1   pound of lean ground pork
1   pound of lean ground beef
2–3 whole bay leaves
1   cup dry red wine
    or low sodium beef broth
2   28-ounce cans of crushed
    plum tomatoes
1   small can of tomato paste,
    plus 1 small can hot water
    Salt and pepper to taste

Put the vegetables into a food processor and process until so fine that it is almost a paste. If you don't have a processor, just chop the vegetables as finely as you can with a large knife.

Sauté the processed vegetables in the olive oil in a large Dutch oven over low heat until golden, about 10 minutes.

Add the meat and continue to use a large spoon to break up the meat as it cooks. When the meat is completely cooked you can drain any excess fat, add the wine or broth, and simmer another 10 minutes.

Add the tomatoes, tomato paste, and water and bring to a full boil. Lower the heat to low and simmer for 3 hours, checking occasionally and adding more water if necessary.

I recommend making the sauce a day ahead, which will improve the flavor and allow you to skim off any fat that hardens on the top of the pot before serving.

Makes approximately 16 (6-ounce or ¾ cup) servings. Each serving counts as 2 lean proteins and 2 vegetables.

Nutrition Facts

Calories 190   Calories from Fat 90

% Daily Value*

	% Daily Value*
Total Fat 10g	15%
Saturated Fat 3g	15%
Trans Fat 0g	
Cholesterol 35mg	12%
Sodium 260mg	11%
Total Carbohydrate 11g	4%
Dietary Fiber 3g	12%
Sugars 2g	
Protein 13g	

Vitamin A 35% • Vitamin C 20%
Calcium 4% • Iron 15%

*Percent Daily Values are based on a 2,000 calorie diet. Your daily values may be higher or lower depending on your calorie needs:

	Calories:	2,000	2,500
Total Fat	Less than	65g	80g
Saturated Fat	Less than	20g	25g
Cholesterol	Less than	300mg	300mg
Sodium	Less than	2,400mg	2,400mg
Total Carbohydrate		300g	375g
Dietary Fiber		25g	30g

Calories per gram:
    Fat 9 • Carbohydrate 4 • Protein 4

Cheesy Waldorf Salad

1 large Granny Smith apple, unpeeled and chopped coarsely
1 tablespoon lemon juice
1 large celery stalk, chopped coarsely
2 tablespoons coarsely chopped walnuts or pecans
2 tablespoons dried cranberries or 20 red grapes cut in half
2 ounces low-fat cheddar cheese, ½-inch dice
2 tablespoons fat-free plain Greek yogurt
1 tablespoon low-fat mayonnaise or salad dressing

Makes 2 servings.
Each serving counts as 1 protein, 1 fat, and 2 fruits.

Keeping your lunches quick, delicious, and exciting doesn't have to be difficult. You can put these salads in small containers to be eaten with a fork, or you can pack a couple of Boston lettuce leaves in a plastic bag and divide the salad portion onto the 2 leaves to make a lettuce wrap at school, at work, on a trip, or at the beach.

Sprinkle the apple chunks with lemon juice and toss (to prevent oxidation and browning).

Add the celery, nuts, fruit, and cheese and toss together.

To make the dressing, whisk the yogurt and mayonnaise together. You can add a sprinkle of cinnamon or apple pie spice or a chopped green herb such as parsley, if you like. Add the dressing to the fruit mixture and toss.

Nutrition Facts		
Calories 220 Calories from Fat 80		
		% Daily Value*
Total Fat 9g		14%
Saturated Fat 2g		10%
Trans Fat 0g		
Cholesterol 5mg		2%
Sodium 260mg		11%
Total Carbohydrate 26g		9%
Dietary Fiber 4g		16%
Sugars 19g		
Protein 10g		
Vitamin A 6%	•	Vitamin C 15%
Calcium 15%	•	Iron 4%

*Percent Daily Values are based on a 2,000 calorie diet. Your daily values may be higher or lower depending on your calorie needs:

		Calories:	2,000	2,500
Total Fat	Less than		65g	80g
Saturated Fat	Less than		20g	25g
Cholesterol	Less than		300mg	300mg
Sodium	Less than		2,400mg	2,400mg
Total Carbohydrate			300g	375g
Dietary Fiber			25g	30g

Calories per gram:
Fat 9 • Carbohydrate 4 • Protein 4

Classic Roasted Chicken

• • • • • • • • • • • • • • • • • • •

I have been watching cooking shows on television since the 1960s when I was a college student mesmerized by Julia Child creating elegant French food. One of the best techniques I learned from Julia was how to roast a chicken. Of course, I have modified the technique using olive oil instead of butter, and my convection oven cooks the chicken faster, but the results are still delicious and the leftovers give me a night off in the kitchen.

1   (3½ to 4 pound) chicken, also known as a "fryer chicken"
2   tablespoons olive oil
1   lemon, quartered (optional)
    Herbs such as rosemary, thyme, or sage (optional)
    Salt and pepper (optional)

Makes 8 (3-ounce) servings (discarded skin and bone is 50 percent of the total weight of the bird, so 1¾ pound of meat is the total yield of a 3½ pound bird). Each serving counts as 3 lean proteins.

Preheat the oven to 425 degrees.

Spray a heavy roasting pan and V-shaped rack with nonstick spray to make clean-up easier.

Remove the chicken from its wrapping and discard the giblets (you may wish to freeze the neck bone for making broth at a later time). Pat the bird dry with a paper towel.

Rub the chicken with olive oil. If desired, stuff the chicken with the quartered lemon and a bunch of herbs to infuse extra flavor. Tie the legs together with cotton cooking twine, and then wrap the twine around the breast, tucking in the wing tips to keep close to the bird. Tie it securely.

Place the chicken on the roasting rack on its side and cook for 15 minutes. Remove the chicken from the oven and turn it on its other side and cook for another 15 minutes. Remove the chicken again from the oven and place it in the breast-up position. At this point you can brush or drizzle another tablespoon of olive oil over the chicken to baste it.

Return the chicken to the oven and roast for approximately another 30 minutes. Total cooking time will depend on the weight of the chicken and your oven.

Using an instant-read thermometer inserted into the middle of the thigh, check to be sure the chicken has reached an internal temperature of 165 degrees.

Cover the roasting pan loosely with a sheet of foil and let the chicken cool for at least 20 minutes before serving. While the chicken is resting, you can cook your vegetables and any other side dishes.

Remove the skin, cut the chicken into 8–12 pieces, and arrange on a platter with lemon wedges and more herbs for garnish.

Nutrition Facts

Calories 110	Calories from Fat 25

% Daily Value*

Total Fat 3g	**5%**
Saturated Fat 1g	**5%**
Trans Fat 0g	
Cholesterol 65mg	**22%**

Sodium 75mg	**3%**
Total Carbohydrate 0g	**0%**
Dietary Fiber 0g	**0%**
Sugars 0g	
Protein 20g	

Vitamin A 0%	•	Vitamin C 4%
Calcium 2%	•	Iron 4%

*Percent Daily Values are based on a 2,000 calorie diet. Your daily values may be higher or lower depending on your calorie needs:

		Calories:	2,000	2,500
Total Fat	Less than		65g	80g
Saturated Fat	Less than		20g	25g
Cholesterol	Less than		300mg	300mg
Sodium	Less than		2,400mg	2,400mg
Total Carbohydrate			300g	375g
Dietary Fiber			25g	30g

Calories per gram:
Fat 9 • Carbohydrate 4 • Protein 4

Curried Scallops

This is the quickest way I know to cook scallops. This method can also be used to cook shrimp. It's a delicious and beautiful way to serve scallops when in season. Be sure to use curry powder that is fresh and full of flavor. Besides imparting a rich flavor to food, curry powder contains curcumin, which has been associated with a lowered risk of Alzheimer's disease.

1 **pound of sea scallops**
1 **tablespoon olive oil**
2–3 **tablespoons curry powder**
   Salt and pepper to taste (optional)

Makes 4 servings.
Each serving counts as
3 lean proteins.

Heat olive oil in a large heavy skillet (preferably well-seasoned black cast iron) over medium high heat.

Sprinkle curry powder in a shallow bowl. Dip the top and bottom of each scallop into the curry powder, shaking off any excess.

Sauté the scallops quickly on each side for just several minutes until cooked through and golden brown. If using smaller bay scallops, sauté for just a couple of minutes shaking the pan occasionally.

Serve these with cooked vegetables, brown rice, or on a bed of mesclun or other greens with a light vinaigrette dressing.

Nutrition Facts		
Calories 130	Calories from Fat 30	
		% Daily Value*
Total Fat 3.5g		5%
Saturated Fat 0g		0%
Trans Fat 0g		
Cholesterol 35mg		12%
Sodium 180mg		8%
Total Carbohydrate 4g		1%
Dietary Fiber 1g		4%
Sugars 0g		
Protein 19g		
Vitamin A 2%	•	Vitamin C 6%
Calcium 4%	•	Iron 6%

*Percent Daily Values are based on a 2,000 calorie diet. Your daily values may be higher or lower depending on your calorie needs:

		Calories:	2,000	2,500
Total Fat	Less than		65g	80g
Saturated Fat	Less than		20g	25g
Cholesterol	Less than		300mg	300mg
Sodium	Less than		2,400mg	2,400mg
Total Carbohydrate			300g	375g
Dietary Fiber			25g	30g

Calories per gram:
Fat 9 • Carbohydrate 4 • Protein 4

Delicata Squash Stuffed with Sausage and Bulgur

● ●

1   **pound apple-smoked chicken sausages, fully cooked, cut in half lengthwise and sliced into ½-inch pieces**
3   **Delicata squash, or small acorn squash**
½   **cup bulgur wheat**
1   **tablespoon olive oil**
1   **small red pepper, cut into ½-inch dice**
1   **small Golden Delicious apple, peeled and cut into ½-inch dice**
1   **clove garlic, minced finely**
    Salt and pepper to taste (optional)
3   **tablespoons maple syrup**
¼   **cup low-fat cheddar cheese, shredded**

Makes 6 servings. Each serving counts as 2 starchy vegetables, 1 whole grain, and 2 proteins.

If you like stuffed peppers, you'll want to try this small squash stuffed with whole-grain bulgur and chicken sausage. The combination of apple and maple with the squash and sausage is a real cool-weather comfort food. Serve with a vegetable soup or a green salad to round out the meal. If using fresh chicken sausage, be sure to cook completely using package directions before adding to the other ingredients.

●

Set the oven to 400 degrees.

Cut each squash in half and remove seeds. Place cut side up in a round glass or ceramic plate and microwave for 10–12 minutes or until the squash is tender. Or you can bake them for 30 minutes in the oven in a roasting pan at 400 degrees.

While the squash is cooking, pour ½ cup of boiling water over the bulgur in 1 medium bowl and let it sit, tightly covered, for 20–30 minutes to absorb the water.

In a large heavy skillet over medium heat, sauté the pepper, apple, and garlic in the olive oil for 2 minutes, stirring occasionally. Add the chicken sausage and continue to cook for another 2 minutes. Add the bulgur and stir to evenly distribute all the components of the stuffing.

When the squash is cooked, drain any water from the pan and turn the squash over with the cut side up. Drizzle ½ tablespoon of maple syrup over each squash, then fill with the stuffing. Top with the shredded cheese and bake for 10–15 minutes or until the cheese has melted.

Nutrition Facts

Calories 310	Calories from Fat 60

	% Daily Value*
Total Fat 7g	**11%**
Saturated Fat 2.5g	**13%**
Trans Fat 0g	
Cholesterol 60mg	**20%**
Sodium 430mg	**18%**
Total Carbohydrate 46g	**15%**
Dietary Fiber 6g	**24%**
Sugars 17g	
Protein 17g	

Vitamin A 30%	•	Vitamin C 70%
Calcium 10%	•	Iron 15%

*Percent Daily Values are based on a 2,000 calorie diet. Your daily values may be higher or lower depending on your calorie needs:

		Calories:	2,000	2,500
Total Fat	Less than		65g	80g
Saturated Fat	Less than		20g	25g
Cholesterol	Less than		300mg	300mg
Sodium	Less than		2,400mg	2,400mg
Total Carbohydrate			300g	375g
Dietary Fiber			25g	30g

Calories per gram:
Fat 9 • Carbohydrate 4 • Protein 4

Five-Spice Pork Pot Roast

Boston butt pork shoulder is not as "neat" as a pork loin but is much tastier. Trimmed of all visible fat and cooked as a pot roast, it is one of the tenderest of meats. It is also one of the most economical cuts of pork, and the leftovers are easily reheated without becoming dry.

Preheat the oven to 325 degrees.

Combine five-spice powder and black pepper in small bowl. Rub the roast all over with the mixture. In a large Dutch oven or covered casserole, heat the oil over medium heat. Brown the pork on all sides until golden brown for approximately 10 minutes, turning every 2–3 minutes to insure all the surface area is seared and sealed to keep the juices in.

Add the garlic to the pan for 1 minute. Pour the beer or broth into the pan and cover tightly. Bake for 3½ to 4½ hours, checking and turning occasionally, adding water if necessary.

Remove the roast from the oven, placing it on a foil-lined roasting pan. Turn the oven up to 450 degrees. Remove the twine from the tied roast. Whisk together the glaze and brush it over the pork. Return to the oven for only 10 minutes. Remove the roast from the oven and place on a platter or cutting board, cover with foil, and let rest for 10–15 minutes to relax the meat and allow the juices to stay in the meat.

6 pound boned and rolled fresh pork shoulder, trimmed of visible fat (5-pound yield)
3 tablespoons Chinese five-spice powder
½ teaspoon ground black pepper
1 teaspoon salt (optional)
2 tablespoons grape seed oil, peanut oil, or canola oil
12 garlic cloves, finely minced
12 ounce light beer or 1½ cups light chicken broth

Glaze

¼ cup tomato ketchup
1 tablespoon dark soy sauce
1 tablespoon Chinese five-spice powder
2 tablespoons brown sugar

Makes 20 servings.
Each serving counts as 3 lean proteins.

Sauce

While the roast is resting, skim excess fat from the pan juices with a large spoon, or you can use a skimming cup (made for just this purpose). Add the remaining glaze and place the casserole or Dutch oven over medium to high heat and reduce the sauce by half (approximately 10 minutes).

Slice or pull the pork apart and serve on a platter. Garnish with orange wedges or herbs.

Meat Only

Nutrition Facts

Calories 180	Calories from Fat 70

% Daily Value*

Total Fat 8g	**12%**
Saturated Fat 3g	**15%**
Trans Fat 0g	
Cholesterol 75mg	**25%**

Sodium 170mg	**7%**
Total Carbohydrate 4g	**1%**
Dietary Fiber 0g	**0%**
Sugars 2g	
Protein 22g	

Vitamin A 0%	•	Vitamin C 2%
Calcium 4%	•	Iron 10%

*Percent Daily Values are based on a 2,000 calorie diet. Your daily values may be higher or lower depending on your calorie needs:

		Calories:	2,000	2,500
Total Fat	Less than		65g	80g
Saturated Fat	Less than		20g	25g
Cholesterol	Less than		300mg	300mg
Sodium	Less than		2,400mg	2,400mg
Total Carbohydrate			300g	375g
Dietary Fiber			25g	30g

Calories per gram:
Fat 9 • Carbohydrate 4 • Protein 4

Sauce Only

Nutrition Facts

Calories 15	Calories from Fat 10

% Daily Value*

Total Fat 1g	**2%**
Saturated Fat 0g	**0%**
Trans Fat 0g	
Cholesterol 0mg	**0%**

Sodium 40mg	**2%**
Total Carbohydrate 1g	**0%**
Dietary Fiber 0g	**0%**
Sugars 1g	
Protein 0g	

Vitamin A 0%	•	Vitamin C 0%
Calcium 0%	•	Iron 0%

*Percent Daily Values are based on a 2,000 calorie diet. Your daily values may be higher or lower depending on your calorie needs:

		Calories:	2,000	2,500
Total Fat	Less than		65g	80g
Saturated Fat	Less than		20g	25g
Cholesterol	Less than		300mg	300mg
Sodium	Less than		2,400mg	2,400mg
Total Carbohydrate			300g	375g
Dietary Fiber			25g	30g

Calories per gram:
Fat 9 • Carbohydrate 4 • Protein 4

Hazelnut-crusted Turkey Burgers

Turkey is so low in fat that adding the beneficial fat in the hazelnuts does not make this recipe as high in calories or fat as you might think. And it's quick and easy to prepare. Even those who complain that turkey is too dry or too boring will fall in love with these burgers.

Buy the blanched nuts that have the skin removed to reduce your preparation time, and store them in the freezer to keep them fresh.

Place the ground turkey in a large bowl.

Using a small food processor, coarsely chop the hazelnuts by pulsing on and off. Add half of the nuts to the bowl. Reserve the other half for coating the burgers.

Individually process the cranberries, onion, celery, and herbs. Add along with the egg to the turkey and mix thoroughly.

Form 6 burgers and place on waxed paper. Sprinkle the remaining chopped hazelnuts onto the top of the burgers. Press the surface lightly to adhere the nuts to the burgers.

Heat a black cast iron griddle or skillet on medium heat. Pour the oil into the heated pan and distribute it around the pan using a spatula, brush, or a paper towel. Add the burgers (nut crust side down) and cook approximately 3 minutes per side or until golden brown, and they have reached an internal temperature of 165 degrees.

1 pound 99% fat-free ground turkey
  cup blanched roasted hazelnuts
2 slices whole-wheat bread, torn into large pieces
¼ cup fresh or frozen cranberries, chopped
¼ cup chopped onion
¼ cup chopped celery
2 tablespoons chopped parsley
½ tablespoon chopped sage or
½ teaspoon dried sage
1 large egg, beaten
  Salt to taste (optional)
1 tablespoon canola oil

Makes 6 (3-ounce) burgers.
Each serving counts as 3 proteins.

Nutrition Facts

Calories 190	Calories from Fat 70	
		% Daily Value*
Total Fat 8g		12%
Saturated Fat 0.5g		3%
Trans Fat 0g		
Cholesterol 65mg		22%
Sodium 100mg		4%
Total Carbohydrate 7g		2%
Dietary Fiber 2g		8%
Sugars 1g		
Protein 22g		
Vitamin A 4%	•	Vitamin C 4%
Calcium 2%	•	Iron 10%

*Percent Daily Values are based on a 2,000 calorie diet. Your daily values may be higher or lower depending on your calorie needs:

		Calories:	2,000	2,500
Total Fat	Less than		65g	80g
Saturated Fat	Less than		20g	25g
Cholesterol	Less than		300mg	300mg
Sodium	Less than		2,400mg	2,400mg
Total Carbohydrate			300g	375g
Dietary Fiber			25g	30g

Calories per gram:
Fat 9 • Carbohydrate 4 • Protein 4

Heavenly Turkey Sandwich

2   slices of Ezekiel 4:9 bread or
    other sprouted bread, toasted
½   clove garlic
2   ounces cooked sliced turkey
    breast
1   small tomato, sliced into 4 slices
½   cup arugula or baby spinach
2   teaspoons extra virgin olive oil

**Makes 1 serving (1 sandwich).
Each serving counts as 2½
lean proteins, 2 whole grains, 1
vegetable, and 1 fat.**

This sandwich deserves the label of heavenly for two reasons. First, it's made with Ezekiel bread, and second, it tastes divine. You can adjust the amount of turkey depending on your protein needs, and you can make it open-face if you want just 1 slice of bread and 1 teaspoon of olive oil. Using sprouted grain bread in this sandwich adds another ounce of plant protein to the sandwich, which makes it heartier and more filling than using bread made from a more refined grain.

Assemble all of the ingredients. Toast the bread, and while it's still hot, rub one toasted side with the half clove of garlic to flavor the bread.

Drizzle a teaspoon of oil on each slice of toast. Then layer the turkey, tomato, and arugula. Press firmly before cutting on the diagonal.

Nutrition Facts

Calories 350   Calories from Fat 100

	% Daily Value*
Total Fat 11g	**17%**
Saturated Fat 1.5g	**8%**
Trans Fat 0g	
Cholesterol 40mg	**13%**
Sodium 500mg	**21%**
Total Carbohydrate 39g	**13%**
Dietary Fiber 7g	**28%**
Sugars 5g	
Protein 24g	

Vitamin A 6%	•	Vitamin C 45%
Calcium 4%	•	Iron 10%

*Percent Daily Values are based on a 2,000 calorie diet. Your daily values may be higher or lower depending on your calorie needs:

		Calories:	2,000	2,500
Total Fat	Less than		65g	80g
Saturated Fat	Less than		20g	25g
Cholesterol	Less than		300mg	300mg
Sodium	Less than		2,400mg	2,400mg
Total Carbohydrate			300g	375g
Dietary Fiber			25g	30g

Calories per gram:
Fat 9 • Carbohydrate 4 • Protein 4

Huevos a la Flamenca

Eggs are one of the most economical and versatile protein sources. This rendition of Spanish Eggs can provide a great brunch dish or a simple supper entrée. In Spain half-portions of this dish (containing a single egg) are often served in cafés as tapas (small plates or snacks). You can use canned tomato sauce instead of making your own, but the sauce recipe below is simple and worth making the night before you need it.

16 ounce can unsalted diced tomatoes
2 tablespoons chopped onions
2 garlic cloves, chopped
1 tablespoon olive oil
1 bay leaf
¼ cup water

Tomato sauce

Sauté the chopped onion and garlic in olive oil for 2–3 minutes over low heat until translucent. Immediately add the diced tomatoes and turn the heat up to medium, stirring or shaking the pan occasionally for 2–3 minutes.

Add the bay leaf and water and bring to a boil. Lower the heat to a simmer and cook for 10–15 minutes to develop the flavor. Cool and remove the bay leaf. You can puree it at this point or use an immersion blender, but I prefer the chunkier consistency.

2 ounces lean boiled ham, chopped into ½-inch dice
8 large eggs
¼ cup cooked green peas
1 roasted red pepper from a jar, drained and sliced into ¼-inch strips
8 spears of asparagus, peeled and cut in thirds lengthwise
2 tablespoons chopped parsley

Eggs

Preheat the oven to 400 degrees.

Spray 4 (10–12 ounce) ramekins with nonstick cooking spray and place them on a small baking sheet. Place 1/4 of the tomato sauce and 1/4 of the ham in each ramekin. Break each egg individually into a custard cup and then add 2 eggs to each ramekin.

Top the eggs with the vegetables and garnish with parsley. Bake for 6–8 minutes or until the whites are set but the yolks are still soft. Remove from the oven and let sit for another minute before serving.

Makes 4 servings.
Each serving counts as 2 vegetables, 2 proteins, and 1 fat.

Nutrition Facts

Calories 240	Calories from Fat 120	
		% Daily Value*
Total Fat 14g		**22%**
Saturated Fat 3.5g		**18%**
Trans Fat 0g		
Cholesterol 430mg		**143%**
Sodium 610mg		**25%**
Total Carbohydrate 10g		**3%**
Dietary Fiber 3g		**12%**
Sugars 6g		
Protein 18g		
Vitamin A 50%	•	Vitamin C 60%
Calcium 8%	•	Iron 20%

*Percent Daily Values are based on a 2,000 calorie diet. Your daily values may be higher or lower depending on your calorie needs:

		Calories:	2,000	2,500
Total Fat	Less than		65g	80g
Saturated Fat	Less than		20g	25g
Cholesterol	Less than		300mg	300mg
Sodium	Less than		2,400mg	2,400mg
Total Carbohydrate			300g	375g
Dietary Fiber			25g	30g

Calories per gram:
Fat 9 • Carbohydrate 4 • Protein 4

Parchment Pesce

- -

1 pound of white fish such as flounder, haddock, halibut, sole, or cod

1 large carrot, cut into matchstick strips

2 large celery stalks, cut into matchstick strips

4 scallions, cut into matchstick strips

2 tablespoons lemon juice

2 tablespoons capers, rinsed and drained

2 teaspoons green peppercorns, rinsed and drained

Makes 4 portions. Each portion counts as 3 lean proteins and 1 vegetable.

Pesce is Italian for fish, and this recipe uses the technique of cooking fish in parchment paper without added fat. Simple elegant cooking makes a small piece of fish go a long way and keeps the cost affordable. I assemble these packets of fish on a rimmed baking sheet an hour or two before my guests arrive, put them in the refrigerator, and then place them in the oven to bake at dinnertime. This is a great entrée for a meal that includes a rich dessert, since the fish is naturally low in fat and this recipe contains no added fat.

Cut parchment paper into 4 sheets approximately 14 x 14 inches. Cut 4 12-inch lengths of white kitchen twine.

Divide the fish into 4 portions and set aside. Mix the matchstick vegetables together in a bowl.

Distribute half the vegetables between the four parchment squares, placing them in the center of the square. Place a fish portion on top of the vegetables and top with the remainder of the vegetables. Top each portion with lemon juice, capers, and peppercorns. You can prepare this without the capers or peppercorns if you like and instead add 2 tablespoons of parsley in its place for color and flavor.

Using the twine and drawing up the parchment over the fish, make a purse shaped package out of each portion. Twist the parchment and tie a bow with twine to seal each package. Place the portions on a rimmed baking sheet. At this point you can refrigerate the packages until you are ready to bake them, if you wish.

Preheat oven to 400 degrees.

Bake for 12–20 minutes depending on the thickness of the fish. Use an instant-read thermometer to be sure that the temperature has reached 145 degrees. You can insert the thermometer right through the parchment to check.

Just before serving, using scissors snip a couple of slits into the top of the parchment. Let each person tear open his or her own portion. Pass a bowl of quinoa, rice, or couscous and add some to the juices that have accumulated around the fish. Enjoy.

Nutrition Facts

Calories 120   Calories from Fat 10

% Daily Value*

Total Fat 1g	**2%**
Saturated Fat 0g	**0%**
Trans Fat 0g	
Cholesterol 65mg	**22%**
Sodium 240mg	**10%**
Total Carbohydrate 5g	**2%**
Dietary Fiber 2g	**8%**
Sugars 2g	
Protein 22g	

Vitamin A 35% • Vitamin C 20%

Calcium 8% • Iron 10%

*Percent Daily Values are based on a 2,000 calorie diet. Your daily values may be higher or lower depending on your calorie needs:

		Calories:	2,000	2,500
Total Fat	Less than	65g	80g
Saturated Fat	Less than	20g	25g
Cholesterol	Less than	300mg	300mg
Sodium	Less than	2,400mg	2,400mg
Total Carbohydrate		300g	375g
Dietary Fiber		25g	30g

Calories per gram:
Fat 9 • Carbohydrate 4 • Protein 4

Portuguese Fish Stew

3 large onions (white, yellow, or red), sliced

3 large cloves garlic, peeled and sliced

3 tablespoons olive oil

3 whole bay leaves

¼ cup Madeira, dry sherry or clam broth

1 16-ounce can unsalted chopped or diced tomatoes

1 large or 2 medium potatoes (peeled and diced)

3 tablespoons chopped flat-leaf parsley

3 whole cloves

¼ teaspoon roasted red pepper flakes (optional)

1 bottle (8 ounces) clam broth (or 1 cup homemade fish stock if you have it)

1 pound of firm white fish (such as cod or halibut)

1 pound of oily fish (such as trout, wild salmon, swordfish or mackerel)

1 teaspoon salt (optional)

Makes 8 servings.
Each serving counts as
3 proteins, 1 vegetable, and
½ starch.

I enjoyed several versions of this stew while traveling along Portugal's coast. Even those who find swordfish or mackerel too strong on their own may like the moist chunks of fish in this dish. You can combine 2 pounds of any available fish or shrimp and it will taste just great. Just don't have swordfish or bluefish more than once a month to avoid consuming too much mercury. Pregnant women should avoid these fish completely and use fish such as haddock or trout. This stew takes 2 hours to cook but it takes only a short active preparation time to assemble. Make this recipe a day ahead and it will be the centerpiece of a quick meal.

Sauté the onions and garlic until just slightly browned, about 10 minutes, in a soup pot or Dutch oven.

Add the bay leaves, wine, tomatoes, potatoes, herbs and spices, clam broth, and 6 cups of water.

Cover and simmer on low heat for about 1 hour. Uncover and simmer another hour. The broth will reduce and become more concentrated.

Cut the fish into 1–2 inch chunks and add to the broth. Simmer only 5–10 minutes or until the fish is just cooked through.

Serve immediately or cover the pot and refrigerate the soup overnight. You can also freeze individual portions at this point, but cool them down in the refrigerator before freezing.

Reheat slowly on top of the stove before serving. Individual portions can be reheated on medium power in your microwave.

Garnish with more parsley or a sprinkle of Parmesan cheese.

Nutrition Facts

Calories 190	Calories from Fat 50	
		% Daily Value*
Total Fat 6g		9%
Saturated Fat 1g		5%
Trans Fat 0g		
Cholesterol 35mg		12%
Sodium 430mg		18%
Total Carbohydrate 14g		5%
Dietary Fiber 2g		8%
Sugars 4g		
Protein 17g		
Vitamin A 8%	•	Vitamin C 25%
Calcium 4%	•	Iron 6%

*Percent Daily Values are based on a 2,000 calorie diet. Your daily values may be higher or lower depending on your calorie needs:

		Calories:	2,000	2,500
Total Fat	Less than		65g	80g
Saturated Fat	Less than		20g	25g
Cholesterol	Less than		300mg	300mg
Sodium	Less than		2,400mg	2,400mg
Total Carbohydrate			300g	375g
Dietary Fiber			25g	30g

Calories per gram:
Fat 9 • Carbohydrate 4 • Protein 4

Quick Black Bean Soup

This quick and easy bean soup can be prepared in about 15 minutes. Keep the nonperishable ingredients in a basket on your shelf and use as an alternative to pizza on a busy night.

Heat olive oil in a 6–8 quart pot or a Dutch oven over medium heat.

Sauté onions until translucent (3–5 minutes). Add garlic and sauté another minute.

Add broth, tomatoes, ketchup, Worcestershire sauce, spices, and beans. Increase the heat to medium high so that the soup comes to a slow boil. When it does, turn the heat down and simmer another 10 minutes.

Add the lime juice just before serving to add a bit of tart flavor and freshness. Season with salt and pepper if desired.

You can serve this as is or garnish with low-fat sour cream or nonfat Greek yogurt, chopped tomatoes, chopped scallions, or low-fat shredded cheese.

2–3 medium onions, chopped (about 2½ cups)
7–8 cloves of garlic, minced or pressed
1 tablespoon olive oil
1 (14½–ounce) can reduced-sodium chicken broth
2 (15-ounce) cans unsalted chopped or chunk tomatoes
2 tablespoons ketchup
2 teaspoons Worcestershire sauce
1½ teaspoons cumin
2 tablespoons olive oil
1–2 tablespoons chili powder (or to taste)
4 (15½–ounce) cans unsalted black beans, drained
2 tablespoons lime juice, or the juice of
1 fresh lime
Salt and pepper to taste (optional)

Makes 8 servings.
Each serving is 2 lean proteins, 3 starches, and 1 vegetable

Nutrition Facts

Calories 290	Calories from Fat 45

	% Daily Value*
Total Fat 5g	8%
Saturated Fat 1g	5%
Trans Fat 0g	
Cholesterol 0mg	0%
Sodium 250mg	10%
Total Carbohydrate 46g	15%
Dietary Fiber 13g	52%
Sugars 7g	
Protein 15g	

Vitamin A 20%	•	Vitamin C 45%
Calcium 15%	•	Iron 25%

*Percent Daily Values are based on a 2,000 calorie diet. Your daily values may be higher or lower depending on your calorie needs:

		Calories:	2,000	2,500
Total Fat	Less than		65g	80g
Saturated Fat	Less than		20g	25g
Cholesterol	Less than		300mg	300mg
Sodium	Less than		2,400mg	2,400mg
Total Carbohydrate			300g	375g
Dietary Fiber			25g	30g

Calories per gram:
Fat 9 • Carbohydrate 4 • Protein 4

Quick Chick Salad

2 cups diced cooked chicken breast
½ medium red onion, diced
1 medium stalk celery, diced
¼ cup chopped red or yellow pepper
¼ cup low-fat mayonnaise
1 tablespoon lemon juice
⅛ teaspoon fresh ground black pepper
1 teaspoon dried dill
8 large leaves of romaine, red-leaf, or Boston lettuce
½ teaspoon paprika
¼ cup chopped parsley

Makes 4 servings.
Each serving counts as 3 lean proteins, 1 vegetable, and 1 fat.

This is a classic lunch choice, and making it with low-fat mayonnaise keeps the salad light on calories. You can also substitute cooked turkey breast for the chicken.

In a medium bowl, combine the chicken and the vegetables.

In a small bowl, combine the mayonnaise, lemon juice, pepper, and dill. Mix or whisk until smooth. Pour into the chicken mixture and toss until the chicken is evenly coated.

You can serve by placing 2 lettuce leaves on 4 plates. Place ¼ of the chicken on each plate. Sprinkle with paprika and parsley before serving.

Nutrition Facts

Calories 180   Calories from Fat 60

	% Daily Value*
Total Fat 7g	11%
Saturated Fat 1g	5%
Trans Fat 0g	
Cholesterol 55mg	18%
Sodium 550mg	23%
Total Carbohydrate 8g	3%
Dietary Fiber 1g	4%
Sugars 3g	
Protein 22g	

Vitamin A 20%   •   Vitamin C 15%
Calcium 4%   •   Iron 8%

*Percent Daily Values are based on a 2,000 calorie diet. Your daily values may be higher or lower depending on your calorie needs:

		Calories:	2,000	2,500
Total Fat	Less than		65g	80g
Saturated Fat	Less than		20g	25g
Cholesterol	Less than		300mg	300mg
Sodium	Less than		2,400mg	2,400mg
Total Carbohydrate			300g	375g
Dietary Fiber			25g	30g

Calories per gram:
Fat 9 • Carbohydrate 4 • Protein 4

Red Chili Con Carne

● ● ● ● ● ● ● ● ● ● ● ● ● ● ● ● ● ● ● ●

I use dark or light red beans, red onion, and tomatoes as the vegetables, but you can vary the type of beans and add zucchini or other vegetables if you like. You can use the leanest ground beef or turkey you can find for the protein.

●

Heat olive oil over medium heat in a Dutch oven or soup pot. Sauté the onion, garlic, and ground meat for approximately 5 minutes. At this point you may want to drain the meat mixture in a sieve to remove additional fat and then return it to the pan.

Mix the chili powder in the boiling water until dissolved. Add to the ground meat mixture. Add the tomatoes, salt, and herbs and cook over very low heat for 30–40 minutes with the cover ajar. Check and stir it every 10 minutes.

Stir in the wine or broth and simmer for 15–20 minutes without the cover, stirring every 5 minutes.

Add the beans and continue to simmer uncovered on low until the beans are hot and the chili is thick, about another 10–15 minutes.

You can make the chili a day ahead but don't add the beans until you reheat it.

2 tablespoons olive oil
1 medium red onion, chopped
2–4 cloves garlic, chopped
1 pound 90–93% ground beef or buffalo (bison), or 99% fat-free ground turkey
¼ cup boiling water
2–3 tablespoons chili powder
1 (28-ounce) can plum tomatoes, including juice
½ teaspoon salt
1½ teaspoon dried basil
1½ teaspoon dried oregano
1 cup dry red wine (or low-sodium beef broth, if you prefer)
2 (15 1/2-ounce) cans red kidney beans, lightly drained

Makes 8 servings.
Each serving counts as 3 proteins, 1 vegetable, and 1 starch.

Chili with Turkey

Nutrition Facts

Calories 220	Calories from Fat 35

	% Daily Value*
Total Fat 4.5g	**7%**
Saturated Fat 0.5g	**3%**
Trans Fat 0g	
Cholesterol 20mg	**7%**

Sodium 650mg	**27%**
Total Carbohydrate 22g	**7%**
Dietary Fiber 6g	**24%**
Sugars 5g	
Protein 21g	

Vitamin A 15%	•	Vitamin C 25%
Calcium 8%	•	Iron 15%

*Percent Daily Values are based on a 2,000 calorie diet. Your daily values may be higher or lower depending on your calorie needs:

		Calories:	2,000	2,500
Total Fat	Less than		65g	80g
Saturated Fat	Less than		20g	25g
Cholesterol	Less than		300mg	300mg
Sodium	Less than		2,400mg	2,400mg
Total Carbohydrate			300g	375g
Dietary Fiber			25g	30g

Calories per gram:
Fat 9 • Carbohydrate 4 • Protein 4

Chili with Beef

Nutrition Facts

Calories 260	Calories from Fat 80

	% Daily Value*
Total Fat 9g	**14%**
Saturated Fat 3g	**15%**
Trans Fat 0g	
Cholesterol 35mg	**12%**

Sodium 660mg	**28%**
Total Carbohydrate 22g	**7%**
Dietary Fiber 6g	**24%**
Sugars 5g	
Protein 19g	

Vitamin A 15%	•	Vitamin C 25%
Calcium 8%	•	Iron 20%

*Percent Daily Values are based on a 2,000 calorie diet. Your daily values may be higher or lower depending on your calorie needs:

		Calories:	2,000	2,500
Total Fat	Less than		65g	80g
Saturated Fat	Less than		20g	25g
Cholesterol	Less than		300mg	300mg
Sodium	Less than		2,400mg	2,400mg
Total Carbohydrate			300g	375g
Dietary Fiber			25g	30g

Calories per gram:
Fat 9 • Carbohydrate 4 • Protein 4

Savory Baked Tilapia

Tilapia is affordable, widely available in markets, and quick to cook. The marinade can be assembled the day or morning before cooking. There's no excuse for not eating more fish when it's this easy and inexpensive. It's great with accompaniments such as rice or polenta and cauliflower, spinach, or green beans.

Rinse and dry tilapia fillets. Place in a rectangular baking dish or glass pie pan.

In a frying pan over medium heat, add olive oil, garlic, onion, oregano, pepper, salt, olives, and tomatoes. Sauté until soft and break up the tomatoes in the pan while cooking. When the onions are soft add the lemon juice and wine or sherry (optional). Keep cooking over medium high heat until the mixture thickens.

Pour the vegetables over the tilapia and allow to marinate for at least 30 minutes.
Preheat oven to 350.
Bake the fish and sauce for 30–40 minutes depending on the thickness of the fillets or until the fish is opaque. Serve immediately.

6   tilapia fillets (4–5 ounces each)
¼   cup lemon juice
¼   cup sherry, white wine, clam or chicken broth
1   teaspoon dried oregano or 1 tablespoon fresh oregano
2   small tomatoes, peeled and chopped (canned is fine)
1   medium yellow onion, cut in half lengthwise and slice thinly
1   medium red onion, cut in half lengthwise and slice thinly
1   tablespoon chopped garlic
½   teaspoon ground black pepper
¼   teaspoon salt (optional)
6   Kalamata olives, pitted and chopped
1   tablespoon olive oil
2   bay leaves

Makes 6 servings.
Each serving counts as 3 proteins and 1 vegetable.

Nutrition Facts

Calories 180	Calories from Fat 50	

	% Daily Value*
Total Fat 6g	9%
Saturated Fat 1g	5%
Trans Fat 0g	
Cholesterol 55mg	18%

Sodium 240mg	10%
Total Carbohydrate 8g	3%
Dietary Fiber 1g	4%
Sugars 3g	
Protein 24g	

Vitamin A 4%	•	Vitamin C 15%
Calcium 2%	•	Iron 4%

*Percent Daily Values are based on a 2,000 calorie diet. Your daily values may be higher or lower depending on your calorie needs:

		Calories:	2,000	2,500
Total Fat	Less than		65g	80g
Saturated Fat	Less than		20g	25g
Cholesterol	Less than		300mg	300mg
Sodium	Less than		2,400mg	2,400mg
Total Carbohydrate			300g	375g
Dietary Fiber			25g	30g

Calories per gram:
Fat 9 • Carbohydrate 4 • Protein 4

Shrimp, Cannellini, and Tomatoes

● ● ● ● ● ● ● ● ● ● ● ● ● ● ● ● ● ● ● ●

¾ pound cooked medium shrimp
1 (16–ounce) can unsalted
   cannellini (white kidney beans),
   rinsed and drained
1 (16–ounce) can unsalted diced
   tomatoes, with juice
1 tablespoon olive oil
2 teaspoons lemon juice
2 tablespoons chopped fresh basil
   or parsley
½ teaspoon red pepper flakes
   (optional)

**Makes 5 servings.
Each serving counts as 3
proteins, 1 starch, and 1
vegetable.**

This dish is a beautiful way to assemble a lunch or dinner without turning on the stove or even the microwave. It's a perfect example of how 3 simple ingredients can be combined to make an elegant and satisfying meal. You can keep the canned goods on hand and some shrimp in the freezer to have ready anytime you need a quick meal.

●

Simply place all ingredients in a large bowl and toss.

This mixture can be served as is at room temperature, chilled on a bed of greens, or heated gently in a pan and served as a stew. You can also enhance it without increasing the calories significantly by adding other vegetables such as zucchini, peppers, cauliflower, broccoli, or onions that have been microwaved, steamed, or roasted.

Nutrition Facts

Calories 210	Calories from Fat 50

	% Daily Value*
Total Fat 6g	9%
Saturated Fat 0.5g	3%
Trans Fat 0g	
Cholesterol 140mg	47%
Sodium 230mg	10%
Total Carbohydrate 16g	5%
Dietary Fiber 4g	16%
Sugars 4g	
Protein 22g	

Vitamin A 20%	•	Vitamin C 35%
Calcium 10%	•	Iron 15%

*Percent Daily Values are based on a 2,000 calorie diet. Your daily values may be higher or lower depending on your calorie needs:

		Calories:	2,000	2,500
Total Fat	Less than		65g	80g
Saturated Fat	Less than		20g	25g
Cholesterol	Less than		300mg	300mg
Sodium	Less than		2,400mg	2,400mg
Total Carbohydrate			300g	375g
Dietary Fiber			25g	30g

Calories per gram:
Fat 9 • Carbohydrate 4 • Protein 4

Smothered Soy Burgers

Frozen soy burgers are a great item to keep on hand for a last-minute meal. They take only a minute or two to microwave or grill. Smothered with caramelized onion and served in an oat-bran pita, they are delicious. Garnish with raw vegetables to complete this fast-food meal.

Sauté the onion slices in a large black cast iron pan or heavy 12-inch skillet over medium low heat, turning often to prevent burning. Cook for 10 minutes or until the onions are wilted and caramelized.

Microwave soy burgers according to package directions. Or you can remove the onions from the skillet and, turning the heat to medium, add the burgers and cook for 1 minute on each side.

Place a burger in each pita half and fill the pocket with the cooked onions. Garnish each with 1 cup raw vegetables.

4　soy burgers
2　large onions,
　　cut into ½-inch slices
1　tablespoon olive oil
2-4　inch whole-grain pitas,
　　sliced in half
2　cups sliced cucumber
1　cup sliced carrot
1　cup sliced radishes

Makes 4 servings.
Each serving counts as 1 whole grain, 3 protein, 2 vegetables, and 1 fat.

Nutrition Facts

Calories 270　Calories from Fat 70

	% Daily Value*
Total Fat 8g	12%
Saturated Fat 0.5g	3%
Trans Fat 0g	
Cholesterol 0mg	0%
Sodium 590mg	25%
Total Carbohydrate 32g	11%
Dietary Fiber 10g	40%
Sugars 7g	
Protein 24g	

Vitamin A 100%　•　Vitamin C 20%
Calcium 4%　•　Iron 6%

*Percent Daily Values are based on a 2,000 calorie diet. Your daily values may be higher or lower depending on your calorie needs:

		Calories:	2,000	2,500
Total Fat	Less than		65g	80g
Saturated Fat	Less than		20g	25g
Cholesterol	Less than		300mg	300mg
Sodium	Less than		2,400mg	2,400mg
Total Carbohydrate			300g	375g
Dietary Fiber			25g	30g

Calories per gram:
Fat 9　•　Carbohydrate 4　•　Protein 4

Steak, Tomatoes, and Artichoke Hearts

● ● ● ● ● ● ● ● ● ● ● ● ● ● ● ● ● ●

½ pound cooked lean
and tender steak (such as
flank steak, beef tenderloin,
or top round)

1 package (10-ounce)
defrosted frozen artichoke hearts
or 1 can (16-ounce) artichoke
hearts, rinsed and drained

4–6 ripe plum tomatoes, seeded and
cut into 6 wedges each

1 large shallot, sliced thin

1 tablespoon extra virgin olive oil

¼ teaspoon dried oregano

⅛ teaspoon crushed red pepper
flakes

8 large Boston or
Bibb lettuce leaves (optional)

Makes 4 servings.
Each serving counts as 2 lean
proteins, 2 vegetables, and 1 fat.

Leftover steak and frozen artichoke hearts can be the basis of a quick lunch or dinner salad. And instead of eating a large steak portion at dinner tonight, slice some of the steak before you sit down to eat and put it into the refrigerator to use for lunch tomorrow. This is a great way to "shrink and multiply" your meals, shrinking your calorie intake and yet enjoying a special treat like steak two days in a row.

●

Slice the steak thinly against the grain. Put in a large bowl.

Cut each artichoke heart into 4 wedges. Add to the steak along with the tomatoes, shallot, olive oil, and seasonings.

The salad can be served on lettuce leaves chilled or at room temperature. It can also be packed in containers to take for lunch. Refrigerate if not using immediately.

Nutrition Facts

Calories 190	Calories from Fat 80

	% Daily Value*
Total Fat 9g	14%
Saturated Fat 2.5g	13%
Trans Fat 0g	
Cholesterol 30mg	10%
Sodium 80mg	3%
Total Carbohydrate 11g	4%
Dietary Fiber 5g	20%
Sugars 3g	
Protein 19g	

Vitamin A 15%	•	Vitamin C 25%
Calcium 4%	•	Iron 10%

*Percent Daily Values are based on a 2,000 calorie diet. Your daily values may be higher or lower depending on your calorie needs:

		Calories:	2,000	2,500
Total Fat	Less than		65g	80g
Saturated Fat	Less than		20g	25g
Cholesterol	Less than		300mg	300mg
Sodium	Less than		2,400mg	2,400mg
Total Carbohydrate			300g	375g
Dietary Fiber			25g	30g

Calories per gram:
Fat 9 • Carbohydrate 4 • Protein 4

Tapenade Tuna

Tapenade is a delicious garnish for a tuna or any fish steak. This recipe makes enough to have some tapenade left over to enjoy on a slice of toasted whole-wheat baguette or whole-grain crackers, or to stuff some cherry tomatoes. Cut the tomatoes in half and scoop out the seeds with a melon ball tool or a grapefruit spoon, then stuff each with 1 teaspoon of tapenade. Because tuna is higher in mercury, eat it only occasionally or reserve this for special treat when fresh tuna is in season.

Make the tapenade by placing the ingredients into the food processor. Pulse several times to chop the ingredients coarsely. Continue to blend until the ingredients are finely minced but not a smooth puree. You want to keep some of the texture of the ingredients.

Prepare the fish by brushing both sides with olive oil. Preheat a black cast iron skillet or a stovetop grill over moderate heat. Add the fish to the hot pan and grill for approximately 4–5 minutes per side if the fish steak is 1 inch thick. Adjust the time depending on the thickness. Check with an instant-read thermometer to make sure the internal temperature is 125 degrees. Remove the fish from the skillet, cover loosely with foil, and allow to sit for 2–3 minutes before serving. Do not overcook or the fish will be dry.

Garnish each portion of the fish steak with 2 tablespoons of the tapenade spooned over the fish.

Tapenade

1   cup pitted Niçoise or Kalamata olives, rinsed and drained
¼   cup capers, rinsed and drained
2   anchovy fillets
    or 2 teaspoons anchovy paste
3   cloves garlic, sliced
2   tablespoons chopped parsley
2   tablespoons lemon juice
⅓   cup extra virgin olive oil

Fish

1   pound fresh tuna, wild salmon steak, or farm-raised trout divided into 4 portions
1   tablespoon olive oil
    Salt and pepper (optional)

Makes 4 servings of tuna and 16 servings of tapenade. Each serving counts as 4 lean proteins and 1 fat.

Tapenade

Nutrition Facts			
Calories 60 Calories from Fat 50	**Sodium** 280mg	**12%**	*Percent Daily Values are based on a 2,000 calorie diet. Your daily values may be higher or lower depending on your calorie needs:
	Total Carbohydrate 1g	**0%**	
% Daily Value*	Dietary Fiber 1g	**4%**	
Total Fat 6g **9%**	Sugars 0g		
Saturated Fat 1g **5%**	**Protein** 0g		
Trans Fat 0g			
Cholesterol 0mg **0%**	Vitamin A 2% • Vitamin C 4%		
	Calcium 2% • Iron 4%		

	Calories:	2,000	2,500
Total Fat	Less than	65g	80g
Saturated Fat	Less than	20g	25g
Cholesterol	Less than	300mg	300mg
Sodium	Less than	2,400mg	2,400mg
Total Carbohydrate		300g	375g
Dietary Fiber		25g	30g
Calories per gram:			
Fat 9 • Carbohydrate 4 • Protein 4			

Tuna

Nutrition Facts			
Calories 190 Calories from Fat 80	**Sodium** 45mg	**2%**	*Percent Daily Values are based on a 2,000 calorie diet. Your daily values may be higher or lower depending on your calorie needs:
	Total Carbohydrate 0g	**0%**	
% Daily Value*	Dietary Fiber 0g	**0%**	
Total Fat 9g **14%**	Sugars 0g		
Saturated Fat 2g **10%**	**Protein** 26g		
Trans Fat 0%			
Cholesterol 45mg **15%**	Vitamin A 50% • Vitamin C 0%		
	Calcium 0% • Iron 6%		

	Calories:	2,000	2,500
Total Fat	Less than	65g	80g
Saturated Fat	Less than	20g	25g
Cholesterol	Less than	300mg	300mg
Sodium	Less than	2,400mg	2,400mg
Total Carbohydrate		300g	375g
Dietary Fiber		25g	30g
Calories per gram:			
Fat 9 • Carbohydrate 4 • Protein 4			

Thin Crust Pizza

Crust

- 1 **cup whole-wheat flour**
- 2 **cups unbleached white flour**
- 1 **teaspoon salt**
- 1 **cup warm water (110–115 degrees)**
- 2½ **teaspoons yeast (1 packet)**
- 1 **tablespoon sugar**
- 3 **tablespoons olive oil**

Making your own pizza is fun for your family and friends and lets you control the type and the amount of cheese, which is the source of most of the calories. The combinations of toppings are endless and the dough is easy to make in a food processor. I often make the dough at breakfast time, cover it with plastic wrap, and place it in the refrigerator until dinner time. Punch down the dough to remove air bubbles and let it come to room temperature before rolling the crust. You can also use 1 pound of purchased pizza dough.

•

Place the flours and the salt in the bowl of a food processor and pulse 3 times. Measure the warm water into a glass measuring cup. Add the sugar and the yeast and stir to dissolve the yeast. Let stand for about 5 minutes.

Add the olive oil and the yeast mixture to the flour and immediately process the dough until it forms a ball, approximately 30 seconds. If the dough is very wet or sticky, you can add 1–3 tablespoons of flour (not too much, because moist dough will be easier to roll into a thin crust). Scrape the dough out of the processor onto a floured surface and knead by hand for 1–2 minutes. Place the dough into an oiled bowl and cover with plastic wrap. Let the dough sit at room temperature for about 45 minutes or until it has doubled in size. Punch down the dough, reshape it into a ball, and return it to the oiled bowl. Cover and place it in the refrigerator.

Place all of the sauce ingredients in a saucepan over moderate heat. Simmer for 15 minutes to develop the flavor and thicken. Cool before making the pizza. You can also use 3 cups of your favorite brand of pizza/pasta sauce in a jar.

Preheat the oven to 425 degrees. If you are using a pizza stone, preheat the oven for at least 20–30 minutes.

To assemble the pizzas, punch down the dough and divide into 2 balls. Roll the dough out thinly, allowing it to rest and relax occasionally during the process. You can roll it out into a round shape for a round pizza pan or stone, or use a rectangular baking sheet.

Ladle about ½ cup or more of sauce onto each pizza. Then top each with half the cheese and half of other vegetables that you have chosen. If you are using dried herbs, sprinkle them onto the pizza before baking. If using fresh herbs, wait until the pizza is done, then garnish.

Bake the pizza for 10–15 minutes or until the crust is golden brown, checking to be sure the bottom of the crust is cooked. Slice and enjoy!

Sauce

- 1 (28-ounce) can unsalted crushed tomatoes
- 2 tablespoons tomato paste
- 2 teaspoons dried or 2 tablespoons fresh chopped basil
- 6 cloves of garlic, finely minced

Toppings

- 12 ounces low-fat shredded Italian-blend cheese or mozzarella
- 8 ounces sliced baby bella mushrooms and/or 2 cups sliced green peppers
- 1 large red or yellow onion, thinly sliced
- ¼ cup pitted black olives, sliced
- 8 cloves garlic
  Other vegetables of your choice, lightly steamed or sautéed (broccoli, asparagus, spinach, artichoke hearts)
  Fresh basil and oregano (or dried herbs)

Makes 2 (16-inch) pizzas, each slice ⅛ of the pizza (16 servings). Each slice is 1 starch, ½ whole grain, 1 protein or high-calcium food, 1 vegetable, 1 fat.

Nutrition Facts

Calories 210	Calories from Fat 60

	% Daily Value*
Total Fat 7g	11%
Saturated Fat 3g	15%
Trans Fat 0g	
Cholesterol 10mg	3%

Sodium 400mg	17%
Total Carbohydrate 27g	9%
Dietary Fiber 3g	12%
Sugars 2g	
Protein 11g	

Vitamin A 15%	•	Vitamin C 10%
Calcium 20%	•	Iron 10%

*Percent Daily Values are based on a 2,000 calorie diet. Your daily values may be higher or lower depending on your calorie needs:

		Calories:	2,000	2,500
Total Fat	Less than		65g	80g
Saturated Fat	Less than		20g	25g
Cholesterol	Less than		300mg	300mg
Sodium	Less than		2,400mg	2,400mg
Total Carbohydrate			300g	375g
Dietary Fiber			25g	30g

Calories per gram:
Fat 9 • Carbohydrate 4 • Protein 4

Triple Bean and Turkey Stew

1   pound lean (93–99%) ground turkey
2   tablespoons olive oil
1   teaspoon smoky chipotle
    seasoning mix
1   teaspoon ground cumin
2   (16-ounce) cans reduced-sodium
    chicken broth
1   teaspoon cider vinegar
1   (16-ounce) can black beans,
    drained and rinsed
1   (16-ounce) can garbanzo beans
    (also known as chickpeas
    or ceci beans), drained and rinsed
3   (16-ounce) cans unsalted diced
    tomatoes, with juice
2   small to medium zucchini,
    cut lengthwise and sliced into
    ½-inch chunks
8   ounces small brown crimini
    mushrooms, halved or quartered
3   garlic cloves, finely minced
¼   teaspoon Tabasco sauce
    (or more to taste)
½   cup kernel corn, frozen or canned
1   red pepper, coarsely chopped
½   cup frozen edamame
    (green soybeans)
1   large sweet potato,
    boiled and mashed

If you're afraid that eating a vegetarian dinner will be too great a shock for you or your family, then try this stew, which gets half of its protein from plant sources and half from the leanest of meats. The stew has a rich flavor and hearty texture that is sure to please even the meat-lovers at your table.

Heat a large Dutch oven or heavy pot over medium heat. Add ground turkey and cook it thoroughly, breaking up the chunks into small pieces as it cooks. Add the seasoning mix and cumin, stirring for 1 minute.

Add the broth and stir. Bring to a boil over medium heat. Add all of the vegetables and beans except the sweet potato. Simmer on low heat for 30 minutes. Add the mashed sweet potato, mixing in thoroughly to blend and form a thick stew. Add another cup of water if the mixture becomes too thick.

Makes 8 servings.
Each serving counts as 1 starchy vegetable, 1 vegetable, and 3 lean proteins.

Nutrition Facts

Calories 290   Calories from Fat 60

% Daily Value*

	% Daily Value*
Total Fat 6g	9%
Saturated Fat 1g	5%
Trans Fat 0g	
Cholesterol 25mg	8%
Sodium 800mg	33%
Total Carbohydrate 36g	12%
Dietary Fiber 11g	44%
Sugars 9g	
Protein 20g	

Vitamin A 130%   •   Vitamin C 70%
Calcium 8%   •   Iron 25%

*Percent Daily Values are based on a 2,000 calorie diet. Your daily values may be higher or lower depending on your calorie needs:

		Calories:	2,000	2,500
Total Fat	Less than		65g	80g
Saturated Fat	Less than		20g	25g
Cholesterol	Less than		300mg	300mg
Sodium	Less than		2,400mg	2,400mg
Total Carbohydrate			300g	375g
Dietary Fiber			25g	30g

Calories per gram:
Fat 9 • Carbohydrate 4 • Protein 4

Turkey Meatballs

These meatballs are just as flavorful as those made with pork and beef. They owe their flavor to the mushrooms and the pine nuts. Freeze the extras in portions for 1 serving or 1 family meal. They can be added to tomato sauce, used in sandwiches, or heated and served plain on a salad.

Sauté the chopped onions in 1 tablespoon olive oil over medium heat, stirring occasionally, for about 6–8 minutes until they are soft but not browned. Let them cool while you are preparing the meat mixture.

Tear the bread slices into a medium bowl and pour the milk over them. Let them absorb the moisture for a few minutes, then pour them into a sieve and press to drain out the excess milk.

In a large bowl combine the turkey, eggs, parsley, porcini mushrooms, and pepper. Mix well with your hands. Add the drained bread, the cooled onions, and the pine nuts and mix thoroughly to distribute the ingredients evenly.

Using a 1-ounce scoop, make rounded balls and place on a sheet pan covered with parchment paper. Once you have portioned out 48 balls, then use your hands to make them round.

At this point you can roll them in flour and sauté them over medium low heat in a heavy skillet in olive oil, or you can bake them in the oven on 2 rimmed baking sheets at 375 degrees for 20–30 minutes.

1   large onion, finely chopped
1   tablespoon olive oil
3   slices whole-wheat or white bread, preferably dry
¾   cup nonfat milk
2½ pounds 99% lean ground turkey
3   eggs, beaten thoroughly
3   tablespoons chopped flat-leaf parsley
⅓   cup dried porcini mushrooms, finely ground in a coffee grinder or food processor
½   teaspoon black pepper
¾   cup lightly roasted pine nuts (pignoli)
2   tablespoons flour
2   tablespoons olive oil for frying

Makes 24 servings (2 meatballs per 2-ounce serving). Each serving counts as 2 proteins.

Sautéed Meatballs

Nutrition Facts

Calories 120   Calories from Fat 40

% Daily Value*

Total Fat 4.5g	7%
Saturated Fat 0.5g	3%
Trans Fat 0g	
Cholesterol 45mg	15%
Sodium 70mg	3%
Total Carbohydrate 6g	2%
Dietary Fiber 3g	12%
Sugars 1g	
Protein 14g	

Vitamin A 2%   •   Vitamin C 2%

Calcium 2%   •   Iron 8%

*Percent Daily Values are based on a 2,000 calorie diet. Your daily values may be higher or lower depending on your calorie needs:

		Calories:	2,000	2,500
Total Fat	Less than		65g	80g
Saturated Fat	Less than		20g	25g
Cholesterol	Less than		300mg	300mg
Sodium	Less than		2,400mg	2,400mg
Total Carbohydrate			300g	375g
Dietary Fiber			25g	30g

Calories per gram:
Fat 9   •   Carbohydrate 4   •   Protein 4

Baked Meatballs

Nutrition Facts

Calories 110   Calories from Fat 30

% Daily Value*

Total Fat 3.5g	5%
Saturated Fat 0g	0%
Trans Fat 0g	
Cholesterol 45mg	15%
Sodium 70mg	3%
Total Carbohydrate 6g	2%
Dietary Fiber 3g	12%
Sugars 1g	
Protein 14g	

Vitamin A 2%   •   Vitamin C 2%

Calcium 2%   •   Iron 8%

*Percent Daily Values are based on a 2,000 calorie diet. Your daily values may be higher or lower depending on your calorie needs:

		Calories:	2,000	2,500
Total Fat	Less than		65g	80g
Saturated Fat	Less than		20g	25g
Cholesterol	Less than		300mg	300mg
Sodium	Less than		2,400mg	2,400mg
Total Carbohydrate			300g	375g
Dietary Fiber			25g	30g

Calories per gram:
Fat 9   •   Carbohydrate 4   •   Protein 4

Whole-grain Grilled Cheese Sandwich

This is an updated version of the classic comfort food sandwich. It is made with whole-grain bread and low-fat cheese and includes a vegetable serving as well as a healthy fat.

Assemble the sandwich.

Heat a heavy skillet using medium low heat. Add olive oil to pan or spray olive oil directly onto one side of the sandwich (place this side down in skillet).

Grill just until the first side starts to turn golden brown. Flip the sandwich and continue to grill for 1–2 more minutes or until the cheese is melted. Cut diagonally into 2 halves.

2 slices sprouted whole-grain bread (such as Ezekiel 4:7 bread or Alvarado Street Bakery bread)
2 (¾-ounce) slices of low-fat cheese (such as light Jarlsberg or 2% American cheese)
1 roasted red pepper (from jar of red peppers packed in water), rinsed and drained
1½ teaspoons olive oil or several sprays of olive oil from an olive oil mister

Makes 2 half-sandwiches.
Each half counts as 1 vegetable, 1 protein, 1 whole grain, and 1 fat.

Nutrition Facts

Calories 200 | Calories from Fat 90

	% Daily Value*
Total Fat 10g	15%
Saturated Fat 4g	20%
Trans Fat 0g	
Cholesterol 15mg	5%
Sodium 320mg	13%
Total Carbohydrate 18g	6%
Dietary Fiber 3g	12%
Sugars 1g	
Protein 10g	

Vitamin A 35% • Vitamin C 35%
Calcium 20% • Iron 6%

*Percent Daily Values are based on a 2,000 calorie diet. Your daily values may be higher or lower depending on your calorie needs:

		2,000	2,500
Total Fat	Less than	65g	80g
Saturated Fat	Less than	20g	25g
Cholesterol	Less than	300mg	300mg
Sodium	Less than	2,400mg	2,400mg
Total Carbohydrate		300g	375g
Dietary Fiber		25g	30g

Calories per gram:
Fat 9 • Carbohydrate 4 • Protein 4

Wild Mushroom Sauté with Whole-grain Pasta

- 3 (8-ounce) packages of wild mushrooms (such as crimini, shitake, oyster, etc.)
- 2 tablespoons olive oil
- 6–8 cloves garlic, peeled and finely chopped
- ½ cup chopped flat-leaf parsley
- 1 cup low-sodium vegetable broth or beef stock
  Fresh ground black pepper to taste
- 8 ounces whole-wheat pasta
- ¾ cup grated Parmesan cheese

Makes 6 servings.
Each serving counts as 2 whole grains, 2 proteins, 2 vegetables, and 1 fat.

The meaty taste of mushrooms is a fitting match for the hearty taste of whole-wheat pasta. The colors of this easy dish are harmonious, as if they were meant to be paired. Garnish with a bit of parsley to complete the earthy flavors. The pasta will cook while you prepare the sauce, so this is a very quick entrée.

Place a large pot of water on high heat and bring to a boil. The pasta will take 8–12 minutes to cook once the water boils, depending on the size of the pasta, so follow package instructions.

Remove any soil or woody stems from the mushrooms. Slice into ½-inch thick slices.

In a large heavy skillet, heat the olive oil over moderate heat. Add garlic and sauté 1–2 minutes, stirring occasionally to prevent burning, before adding the mushrooms.

Sauté the mushrooms for at least 10 minutes to ensure that the moisture in the mushrooms has evaporated and that the mushrooms are browned. Add the broth and cook for another 3 minutes. Turn off heat.

Drain the cooked pasta and add it to the mushroom mixture along with the chopped parsley. Toss and serve. Sprinkle 2 tablespoons of cheese on each serving. Garnish with a sprig of parsley.

Nutrition Facts

Calories 260   Calories from Fat 80

	% Daily Value*
Total Fat 8g	12%
Saturated Fat 2g	10%
Trans Fat 0g	
Cholesterol 5mg	2%
Sodium 200mg	8%
Total Carbohydrate 35g	12%
Dietary Fiber 6g	24%
Sugars 3g	
Protein 14g	

Vitamin A 8% • Vitamin C 15%
Calcium 20% • Iron 15%

*Percent Daily Values are based on a 2,000 calorie diet. Your daily values may be higher or lower depending on your calorie needs:

		Calories:	2,000	2,500
Total Fat	Less than		65g	80g
Saturated Fat	Less than		20g	25g
Cholesterol	Less than		300mg	300mg
Sodium	Less than		2,400mg	2,400mg
Total Carbohydrate			300g	375g
Dietary Fiber			25g	30g

Calories per gram:
Fat 9 • Carbohydrate 4 • Protein 4

Asian Slaw

• •

I like to make this with green and red cabbage, but any variety or combination of cabbages will do. The dressing is flavorful and lower in calories than mayonnaise or traditional cole slaw dressing.

•

Toss the vegetables together in a large bowl. Whisk the dressing ingredients together and pour over the slaw. Toss together until the dressing is fully incorporated. Chill for 30 minutes before serving.

Vegetables

½   **medium head of cabbage, shredded (about 5 cups)**
2   **bunches scallions, sliced very thinly on the diagonal**
½   **cup snow peas, sliced very thinly on the diagonal**
½   **cup shredded carrots**
½   **cup sweet red peppers, cut into matchstick strips**

Dressing

2   **tablespoons low-sodium soy sauce**
1   **tablespoon mirin (sweet rice wine) or sherry (optional)**
1   **tablespoon rice vinegar**
2   **teaspoons toasted sesame oil (or use chili oil if you want it spicy)**
1   **tablespoon toasted sesame seeds**
1   **tablespoon grated fresh ginger root**
2   **teaspoons sugar**

**Makes 12 (½-cup) servings.
Each serving counts as
1 vegetable.**

Nutrition Facts

Calories 45   Calories from Fat 10

                 % Daily Value*

Total Fat 1g	**2%**
Saturated Fat 0g	**0%**
Trans Fat 0g	
Cholesterol 0mg	**0%**
Sodium 80mg	**3%**
Total Carbohydrate 7g	**2%**
Dietary Fiber 2g	**8%**
Sugars 4g	
Protein 1g	

Vitamin A 25%   •   Vitamin C 60%
Calcium 4%   •   Iron 10%

*Percent Daily Values are based on a 2,000 calorie diet. Your daily values may be higher or lower depending on your calorie needs:

		Calories:	2,000	2,500
Total Fat	Less than		65g	80g
Saturated Fat	Less than		20g	25g
Cholesterol	Less than		300mg	300mg
Sodium	Less than		2,400mg	2,400mg
Total Carbohydrate			300g	375g
Dietary Fiber			25g	30g

Calories per gram:
  Fat 9   •   Carbohydrate 4   •   Protein 4

Asparagus on Toast with Mock Hollandaise Sauce

• • • • • • • • • • • • • • • • • • •

1   pound asparagus
4   slices whole-grain bread for
     toasting

Mock Hollandaise

⅓   cup liquid egg substitute
1½   tablespoons butter
1½   teaspoons lemon juice
¾   teaspoon Dijon mustard
     Dash of ground cayenne pepper

Makes 4 servings.
Each serving counts as 1 whole
grain, 1 protein, 1 vegetable, and
½ fat.

One of my favorite breakfasts as a child was asparagus on toast with cheese. This is a healthier and more sophisticated version that is a treat on a weekend. It's easy to make and the whole-grain toast contributes flavor and fiber. Of course, you can substitute a slice of low-fat cheese for the sauce for a super-quick start to the day. Just place the cheese on the warm toast and top with the warm asparagus and it will melt.

•

Peel the asparagus stalks if they are thick or tough. Break off the tough ends of the stalks and arrange the spears in a nonreactive dish (a glass pie plate is good) with the tips toward the middle. Microwave for 5–8 minutes on high but check every 2 minutes to make sure the asparagus retains some crispness. The cooking process will continue for 2 minutes after you remove it from the microwave.

Toast the whole-grain bread and put each slice on a plate.

To make the sauce, pour the egg substitute into a 1-cup glass measuring pitcher. Add the butter. Microwave on 20% power for 30 seconds; stir and continue cooking for another 30 seconds until the butter is melted.

Stir the lemon juice and mustard into the egg mixture and microwave on 20% power for another 3–4 minutes, stirring every 30 seconds until the mixture is thickened. Stir in the cayenne pepper. Use an immersion blender or beat with a wire whisk briefly if the sauce curdles.

Assemble the dish by dividing the asparagus between 4 slices of toast. Top with sauce.

Nutrition Facts

Calories 140	Calories from Fat 50

	% Daily Value*
Total Fat 5g	8%
Saturated Fat 3g	15%
Trans Fat 0g	
Cholesterol 10mg	3%
Sodium 230mg	10%
Total Carbohydrate 16g	5%
Dietary Fiber 4g	16%
Sugars 3g	
Protein 9g	

Vitamin A 30%	•	Vitamin C 15%
Calcium 6%	•	Iron 10%

*Percent Daily Values are based on a 2,000 calorie diet. Your daily values may be higher or lower depending on your calorie needs:

		Calories:	2,000	2,500
Total Fat	Less than		65g	80g
Saturated Fat	Less than		20g	25g
Cholesterol	Less than		300mg	300mg
Sodium	Less than		2,400mg	2,400mg
Total Carbohydrate			300g	375g
Dietary Fiber			25g	30g

Calories per gram:
Fat 9 • Carbohydrate 4 • Protein 4

Basic Green Salad and Vinaigrette

• • • • • • • • • • • • • • • • • • •

In my kitchen salads vary by the season and the availability of the type of greens. Although many green leafy vegetables are available year round today, those that are in season are often fresher, less expensive, and more flavorful. Summer greens such as Boston lettuce, romaine, or leaf lettuces also work well with the lightness of this dressing. Winter leafy vegetables such as escarole, chicory, radicchio, or red cabbage blend well with red wine vinegar in this simple dressing.

Place vinegar or lemon juice, water, and olive oil in a large metal or glass bowl. Whisk these together until they thicken (about 30 seconds). Add salt and pepper if desired.

Toss the greens to coat thoroughly with dressing.

Vary the flavor by adding one of the optional ingredients above. You can also vary the flavor by substituting balsamic vinegar, red wine vinegar, champagne or other vinegars, and even other juices such as orange or lime juice. By using different oils such as avocado oil, walnut oil, or grape seed oil you can achieve an endless variety of flavors from these ingredients.

Add additional vegetables, beans, chickpeas, edamame, or fruits for added nutrition and taste.

8 cups coarsely chopped mixed greens or field greens
1 tablespoon rice vinegar or lemon juice
2½ tablespoons olive oil
2 teaspoons water
Pinch of salt (optional) and ground black pepper

Options to add: 2 minced garlic cloves, 1 teaspoon anchovy paste, 2 teaspoons Dijon mustard, 2 teaspoons Parmesan cheese, 1–2 teaspoons chopped fresh herbs (or half as much dried)

Makes 4 servings.
Each serving counts as 2 vegetables and 2 fats.

Nutrition Facts

Calories 100 Calories from Fat 80

% Daily Value*

Total Fat 9g	14%
Saturated Fat 1g	5%
Trans Fat 0g	
Cholesterol 0mg	0%
Sodium 40mg	2%
Total Carbohydrate 5g	2%
Dietary Fiber 3g	12%
Sugars 3g	
Protein 1g	

Vitamin A 80% • Vitamin C 0%
Calcium 0% • Iron 6%

*Percent Daily Values are based on a 2,000 calorie diet. Your daily values may be higher or lower depending on your calorie needs:

		Calories:	2,000	2,500
Total Fat	Less than		65g	80g
Saturated Fat	Less than		20g	25g
Cholesterol	Less than		300mg	300mg
Sodium	Less than		2,400mg	2,400mg
Total Carbohydrate			300g	375g
Dietary Fiber			25g	30g

Calories per gram:
Fat 9 • Carbohydrate 4 • Protein 4

Green Beans and Shallots

1 pound fresh green beans, stems removed
1–2 shallots, peeled and thinly sliced
½ teaspoon salt
1 tablespoon olive oil
Salt and pepper to taste (optional)

Makes 8 servings.
Each serving counts as 1 vegetable.

Adding a layer of flavor to ordinary vegetables can increase their acceptance by unenthusiastic eaters. Shallots are now available in most supermarkets and give a flavor that is similar to garlic or red onion but is much milder. These green beans are delicious hot or at room temperature, so they're great for a company meal since you can cook them before your guests arrive. And you can save any extra for a great lunch side dish with some cooked chicken.

Bring a large saucepan of water to a full boil and add salt. This will keep the green beans from turning gray, and very little is absorbed into the beans.

Add the beans and cook for only 3–5 minutes, tasting to see if they are still a little crunchy; they will cook further in the skillet, so you don't want them to be overcooked at this stage of the preparation. Drain them into a colander, add 8–10 ice cubes, and run cold water over them to cool the beans and retain their bright green color. When completely drained, dry them with a clean kitchen towel or paper towels.

Heat a large skillet over moderate heat. Add the olive oil and then the shallots and cook for 2–3 minutes until golden brown. Add the green beans and cook for another 3–5 minutes. Serve hot or at room temperature.

Nutrition Facts		
Calories 40	Calories from Fat 15	
		% Daily Value*
Total Fat 2g		3%
Saturated Fat 0g		0%
Trans Fat 0g		
Cholesterol 0mg		0%
Sodium 0mg		0%
Total Carbohydrate 6g		2%
Dietary Fiber 2g		8%
Sugars 2g		
Protein 1g		
Vitamin A 2%	•	Vitamin C 8%
Calcium 2%	•	Iron 2%

*Percent Daily Values are based on a 2,000 calorie diet. Your daily values may be higher or lower depending on your calorie needs:

	Calories:	2,000	2,500
Total Fat	Less than	65g	80g
Saturated Fat	Less than	20g	25g
Cholesterol	Less than	300mg	300mg
Sodium	Less than	2,400mg	2,400mg
Total Carbohydrate		300g	375g
Dietary Fiber		25g	30g

Calories per gram:
Fat 9 • Carbohydrate 4 • Protein 4

Lemon-marinated Vegetables

Making vegetables in advance is the surest way to have them readily available for a snack or a meal. The only cooking involved in this recipe is cooking the carrots. The marinade does the rest of the work. You can prepare these at breakfast time and they will be ready for dinner tonight.

Place the carrots and ¼ cup water in a covered glass dish and microwave on high for 5–8 minutes or until barely tender (times vary with the power level of the microwave). Drain and cool.

In the meantime place the mushrooms and peppers in a large glass container or large zipper-type plastic bag. Add the cooled carrots.

In a small bowl, zest the lemon and squeeze the juice. Add the rest of the ingredients, mix, and pour over the vegetables. Stir to coat all the vegetables.

3 cups of carrots, sliced ½-inch thick on the diagonal
8 ounce package of small button mushrooms
1 small red pepper, cut into 1-inch chunks
1 small yellow or orange pepper, cut into 1-inch chunks
1 lemon, zest and juice
1 teaspoon sugar
1 tablespoon extra virgin olive oil
2 cloves garlic, finely minced (optional)
½ teaspoon dried basil leaves
½ teaspoon dried oregano
¼ teaspoon fresh ground black pepper

Makes 8 servings.
Each serving counts as
1 vegetable.

Nutrition Facts

Calories 35	Calories from Fat 10

% Daily Value*

Total Fat 1g	2%
Saturated Fat 0g	0%
Trans Fat 0g	
Cholesterol 0mg	0%
Sodium 20mg	1%
Total Carbohydrate 6g	2%
Dietary Fiber 2g	8%
Sugars 3g	
Protein 1g	

Vitamin A 110% • Vitamin C 45%
Calcium 2% • Iron 2%

*Percent Daily Values are based on a 2,000 calorie diet. Your daily values may be higher or lower depending on your calorie needs:

		Calories:	2,000	2,500
Total Fat	Less than		65g	80g
Saturated Fat	Less than		20g	25g
Cholesterol	Less than		300mg	300mg
Sodium	Less than		2,400mg	2,400mg
Total Carbohydrate			300g	375g
Dietary Fiber			25g	30g

Calories per gram:
Fat 9 • Carbohydrate 4 • Protein 4

Marinated Cauliflower

Vegetables

1 large head of cauliflower, cored and cut into 1-inch florets
½ cup pitted and sliced Kalamata olives, rinsed
1 bunch scallions, cut into ½-inch slices
½ cup coarsely chopped flat-leaf parsley

Marinade

¼ cup extra virgin olive oil
2 tablespoons red wine vinegar
1½ tablespoons Dijon mustard
1 tablespoon water

Makes 12 (½-cup) servings. Each serving counts as 1 vegetable and 1 fat.

Prepare this vegetable dish tonight while you are making dinner. Let it marinate overnight to absorb all of the flavors and it will taste even better tomorrow. Serve it as a side dish or add it to a green salad. It keeps well for 3 days, so you can portion some into small containers for lunch during the week.

Microwave the cauliflower florets for just 1 minute. Let cool and place in a large bowl.

Add the olives, scallions, and parsley to the cauliflower.

Wisk the marinade ingredients together and pour over the vegetables. Toss so that the marinade coats the cauliflower evenly. Refrigerate overnight. Toss again before serving.

Nutrition Facts

Calories 80	Calories from Fat 60	
		% Daily Value*
Total Fat 7g		11%
Saturated Fat 1g		5%
Trans Fat 0g		
Cholesterol 0mg		0%
Sodium 180mg		8%
Total Carbohydrate 6g		2%
Dietary Fiber 2g		8%
Sugars 2g		
Protein 2g		
Vitamin A 8%	•	Vitamin C 60%
Calcium 4%	•	Iron 4%

*Percent Daily Values are based on a 2,000 calorie diet. Your daily values may be higher or lower depending on your calorie needs:

		Calories:	2,000	2,500
Total Fat	Less than		65g	80g
Saturated Fat	Less than		20g	25g
Cholesterol	Less than		300mg	300mg
Sodium	Less than		2,400mg	2,400mg
Total Carbohydrate			300g	375g
Dietary Fiber			25g	30g

Calories per gram:
Fat 9 • Carbohydrate 4 • Protein 4

Minted Pea Soup

● ●

Treat your taste buds with this fresh version of pea soup without the ham. It has lots of fiber and is a great first course instead of a salad. The mint gives it fresh-from-the-garden spring flavor.

In a large saucepan or small stockpot, heat 2 tablespoons olive oil. Add the chopped vegetables and cook for 10 minutes over medium-low heat until they are soft but not browned.

Turn the heat to high. Add the broth and bring it to a boil, then add the frozen peas and cook for 2–4 minutes. Add more broth or water if necessary to make 2 quarts total.

Turn off the heat and add the mint, salt, and pepper.

Using a handheld immersion blender, puree the soup until smooth. Or place half the batch of soup into a traditional blender and process until smooth. Repeat with remaining half.

Return the soup to low heat to make sure it's hot before serving.

Garnish with a tablespoon of low-fat sour cream and long stems of fresh chives draped across the bowl.

2   tablespoons light olive oil or grape seed oil
1   large Vidalia onion, chopped coarsely
2   leeks, chopped coarsely
2   (16–ounce) cans light chicken broth (or 4 cups homemade chicken broth)
1   (16–ounce) bag of frozen peas (3–4 cups)
2   tablespoons dried chopped mint or ½ cup chopped fresh mint (tightly packed)
½   teaspoon ground white pepper
½   teaspoon salt (optional)

Makes 8 (1-cup) servings. Each serving counts as 1 vegetable, 1 starchy vegetable, and 1 fat.

Nutrition Facts

Calories 100   Calories from Fat 30

	% Daily Value*
Total Fat 4g	**6%**
Saturated Fat 0.5g	**3%**
Trans Fat 0g	
Cholesterol 0mg	**0%**
Sodium 270mg	**11%**
Total Carbohydrate 14g	**5%**
Dietary Fiber 4g	**16%**
Sugars 5g	
Protein 4g	

Vitamin A 30%	•	Vitamin C 20%
Calcium 4%	•	Iron 8%

*Percent Daily Values are based on a 2,000 calorie diet. Your daily values may be higher or lower depending on your calorie needs:

		Calories:	2,000	2,500
Total Fat	Less than		65g	80g
Saturated Fat	Less than		20g	25g
Cholesterol	Less than		300mg	300mg
Sodium	Less than		2,400mg	2,400mg
Total Carbohydrate			300g	375g
Dietary Fiber			25g	30g

Calories per gram:
Fat 9 • Carbohydrate 4 • Protein 4

Orange-glazed Carrots

• •

1 **pound carrots
   (preferably of similar size)
   Zest of ½ orange
   Juice of ½ orange**
2 **teaspoons honey**

**Makes 4 servings.
Each serving counts as 2
vegetables.**

This dish is a child-friendly vegetable that adults will also enjoy. It goes with virtually any kind of fish, poultry, and meat or soy protein. Make a double batch and use the leftovers to enhance a salad or as a second vegetable tomorrow night.

Wash and peel carrots. Slice on the diagonal about ¼-inch thick. Place in a medium-size nonreactive covered dish suitable for microwaving.

Add the orange zest, orange juice, and honey to the carrots and toss.

Cover the dish and microwave on high for 3–4 minutes. Stir. Microwave for an additional 2–3 minutes or until the carrots are crisp-tender.

Transfer carrots and liquid to a medium skillet and turn the heat on medium-high. Cook until the glaze forms (1–2 minutes), stirring or shaking the pan to prevent scorching or sticking.

Nutrition Facts

Calories 50	Calories from Fat 0

% Daily Value*

Total Fat 0g	**0%**
Saturated Fat 0g	**0%**
Trans Fat 0g	
Cholesterol 0mg	**0%**
Sodium 60mg	**3%**
Total Carbohydrate 12g	**4%**
Dietary Fiber 3g	**12%**
Sugars 6g	
Protein 1g	

Vitamin A 360%	•	Vitamin C 15%	
Calcium 4%	•	Iron 2%	

*Percent Daily Values are based on a 2,000 calorie diet. Your daily values may be higher or lower depending on your calorie needs:

		Calories:	2,000	2,500
Total Fat	Less than		65g	80g
Saturated Fat	Less than		20g	25g
Cholesterol	Less than		300mg	300mg
Sodium	Less than		2,400mg	2,400mg
Total Carbohydrate			300g	375g
Dietary Fiber			25g	30g

Calories per gram:
    Fat 9 • Carbohydrate 4 • Protein 4

Roasted Roots

• •

Root vegetables often don't get the respect they deserve, so here's a recipe that can renew your appreciation of them. They have a natural sweetness that is beautifully balanced by a drizzle of balsamic vinegar after cooking.

•

Preheat oven to 400 degrees.

Cut all of the vegetables into 1-inch chunks unless they are already small, such as garlic cloves, small onions, and shallots. These can be left whole. This step can be done ahead and the vegetables stored in the refrigerator for up to 3 days prior to cooking.

Place the vegetable chunks into a large heavy roasting pan and spray or drizzle with the olive oil. Toss to coat the vegetables evenly.

Roast for 20 minutes. Stir with spatula and return to oven for another 15–20 minutes or until golden brown. Sprinkle with vinegar and herbs and toss before serving.

6   cups of mixed root vegetables (including beets, carrots, celeriac, garlic, kohlrabi, onions, parsnips, rutabaga, shallots, sweet potatoes, or turnips)
2   tablespoons extra virgin olive oil
2   tablespoons balsamic vinegar
¼   cup basil or parsley for garnish

Makes 6 servings.
Each serving counts as 1 starchy vegetable, 1 vegetable, and 1 fat.

Nutrition Facts

Calories 130	Calories from Fat 45

	% Daily Value*
Total Fat 5g	8%
Saturated Fat 0.5g	3%
Trans Fat 0g	
Cholesterol 0mg	0%
Sodium 100mg	4%
Total Carbohydrate 20g	7%
Dietary Fiber 3g	12%
Sugars 9g	
Protein 3g	

Vitamin A 160%	•	Vitamin C 35%
Calcium 4%	•	Iron 8%

*Percent Daily Values are based on a 2,000 calorie diet. Your daily values may be higher or lower depending on your calorie needs:

		Calories:	2,000	2,500
Total Fat	Less than		65g	80g
Saturated Fat	Less than		20g	25g
Cholesterol	Less than		300mg	300mg
Sodium	Less than		2,400mg	2,400mg
Total Carbohydrate			300g	375g
Dietary Fiber			25g	30g

Calories per gram:
    Fat 9 • Carbohydrate 4 • Protein 4

Roasted Summer Vegetables

2–3 **bell peppers of different colors**
2 **small or 1 large summer squash**
2 **small or 1 large zucchini**
2 **small or 1 large fennel bulb (or use a total of 8 cups chunked summer vegetables and onions)**
2 **tablespoons olive oil**
½ **cup chopped fresh parsley or basil, or 2–3 tablespoons balsamic vinegar (garnish)**

Makes 6 servings. Each serving counts as 2 vegetable servings and 1 fat.

Vegetables don't have to be boiled and boring. Try these simple roasted vegetables tonight for dinner or make the recipe in advance and portion it into containers of individual servings to have ready for lunch or a snack. It works well for a busy weeknight if you cut up the vegetables in advance, store in a container or bag, and then just sprinkle with olive oil and put in the oven to cook. These vegetables also can be used as a pasta topping.

Preheat oven to 450 degrees.

Clean and remove seeds and white membrane from peppers. Cut into large chunks (approximately 1½ to 2 inches) and add to a large roasting pan.

Cut summer squash and zucchini into halves lengthwise. If they are large, cut them again into quarters lengthwise. Cut these into 1½-inch chunks and add to the pan.

Cut the dark green tops off the fennel; cut in 4 wedges and remove core; cut each quarter into chunks the size of the other vegetables.

Drizzle with 2 tablespoons olive oil and roast for 10–15 minutes. The vegetables should be starting to brown. With a spatula, turn the vegetables over and roast for another 10–15 minutes, until well caramelized. Garnish with parsley, basil, or balsamic vinegar. Enjoy hot, cold, or at room temperature.

Nutrition Facts

Calories 80	Calories from Fat 45

	% Daily Value*
Total Fat 5g	8%
Saturated Fat 0.5g	3%
Trans Fat 0g	
Cholesterol 0mg	0%
Sodium 25mg	1%
Total Carbohydrate 9g	3%
Dietary Fiber 3g	12%
Sugars 3g	
Protein 2g	

Vitamin A 10%	•	Vitamin C 130%
Calcium 4%	•	Iron 4%

*Percent Daily Values are based on a 2,000 calorie diet. Your daily values may be higher or lower depending on your calorie needs:

		Calories:	2,000	2,500
Total Fat	Less than		65g	80g
Saturated Fat	Less than		20g	25g
Cholesterol	Less than		300mg	300mg
Sodium	Less than		2,400mg	2,400mg
Total Carbohydrate			300g	375g
Dietary Fiber			25g	30g

Calories per gram:
Fat 9 • Carbohydrate 4 • Protein 4

Sesame Asparagus

This interesting, Asian-inspired vegetable combination can be made in advance and packaged to go for a great lunch item or snack. You can use fresh asparagus, fresh or frozen green beans, or broccoli.

Steam the vegetables in ½-inch boiling water for 2–3 minutes. Transfer the vegetables to a colander and then plunge it into cold water with a few ice cubes. Drain well and place in a storage container. Add other ingredients and toss to coat the vegetables evenly.

1½ pounds asparagus, green beans, or broccoli, washed and trimmed

1 teaspoon dark toasted sesame oil
A few drops hot chili oil (optional)

1 teaspoon rice vinegar

2–3 tablespoons toasted sesame seeds (a small handful)
Coarse salt (optional)

Makes 6 servings.
Each serving counts as 1 vegetable.

Nutrition Facts			
Calories 30	Calories from Fat 10		
	% Daily Value*		
Total Fat 1g	2%		
Saturated Fat 0g	0%		
Trans Fat 0g			
Cholesterol 0mg	0%		
Sodium 15mg	1%		
Total Carbohydrate 4g	1%		
Dietary Fiber 2g	8%		
Sugars 1g			
Protein 3g			
Vitamin A 20%	• Vitamin C 15%		
Calcium 2%	• Iron 6%		

*Percent Daily Values are based on a 2,000 calorie diet. Your daily values may be higher or lower depending on your calorie needs:

		Calories:	2,000	2,500
Total Fat	Less than	65g	80g
Saturated Fat	Less than	20g	25g
Cholesterol	Less than	300mg	300mg
Sodium	Less than	2,400mg	2,400mg
Total Carbohydrate		300g	375g
Dietary Fiber		25g	30g

Calories per gram:
Fat 9 • Carbohydrate 4 • Protein 4

Shades of Red Salad

• •

4   red, orange, or variegated red-
    orange beets
2   tablespoons light olive oil
¼   teaspoon salt (optional)
¼   teaspoon ground black pepper
    Juice of ½ blood orange
2   teaspoons molasses
    (pomegranate molasses is
    preferable) or honey
1   tablespoon white wine vinegar,
    or champagne vinegar
1   medium red onion,
    sliced very thin
2–3 blood oranges, peeled and cut
    into wedges or thin slices
    Seeds from 1 pomegranate
    (optional)

Makes 4 servings.
Each serving counts as
1 vegetable, 1 fruit, and 1 fat.

Combine fruits and vegetables of the winter season for a delicious, colorful, and nutritionally rich first course or side dish for your holiday table. Pomegranates are one of the foods highest in antioxidants. They are an ancient food mentioned in the Bible, and they remain part of the cuisine of France, Italy, Iran, Morocco, and California, where they are now grown. Blood oranges are named for the unusual red color of their pulp.

Preheat oven to 400 degrees. Wrap beets in foil and roast until beets are tender, approximately 1 hour. Open foil to cool beets. When cool, peel beets and cut each into at least 8 wedges or slices.

In a large bowl whisk blood orange juice, molasses or honey, vinegar, and oil. Season with pepper and salt (optional). Add beet wedges, onion slices, orange sections, and pomegranate seeds. Toss and check for seasoning. Serve on leaves of red leaf or Boston lettuce.

Nutrition Facts		
Calories 120 Calories from Fat 40		
		% Daily Value*
Total Fat 5g		8%
Saturated Fat 0.5g		3%
Trans Fat 0g		
Cholesterol 0mg		0%
Sodium 50mg		2%
Total Carbohydrate 18g		6%
Dietary Fiber 4g		16%
Sugars 12g		
Protein 2g		
Vitamin A 50%	•	Vitamin C 70%
Calcium 6%	•	Iron 6%

*Percent Daily Values are based on a 2,000 calorie diet. Your daily values may be higher or lower depending on your calorie needs:

		Calories:	2,000	2,500
Total Fat	Less than		65g	80g
Saturated Fat	Less than		20g	25g
Cholesterol	Less than		300mg	300mg
Sodium	Less than		2,400mg	2,400mg
Total Carbohydrate			300g	375g
Dietary Fiber			25g	30g

Calories per gram:
Fat 9 • Carbohydrate 4 • Protein 4

Stuffed Roasted Onions

This dish is easy to make for a crowd or for just two. It's elegant enough to serve for a special occasion or a holiday. The butternut squash provides the starch, so I recommend serving this with green beans or Brussels sprouts. What a way to eat your veggies!

Preheat the oven to 425 degrees.

Cut off the root end of the onions so that they will be stable in the roasting pan. Discard the ends. Cut another ¾ to 1 inch from the stem end of the onions. Peel and chop these ends and set aside.

Brush the prepared onions with 2 tablespoons of olive oil and place them root end up in a heavy roasting pan. Roast them for 1 hour or more (depending on the size) until they are soft when pierced with a paring knife.

While the onions are roasting, heat the remaining 1 tablespoon of oil in a skillet. Add the chopped bits of onions and cook them over medium heat until golden brown. Add them to the mashed squash and mix well. Keep warm until you are ready to stuff the onions.

Cool the roasted onions until you can handle them easily to remove the outer skin layers and 1–2 inches of the center of each onion. Preheat the broiler. Stuff each onion with about ½ cup of mashed butternut squash. Broil for a couple of minutes until the tops are golden brown.

These can be prepared in advance and broiled just before serving. Simply place the onions in a 350-degree oven for 20 minutes to warm them and then proceed to the broiling. You can also microwave leftovers another night and they will taste even better.

Save any extra mashed butternut squash for another meal.

8   large (8-ounce) Vidalia onions
1   (2-pound) butternut squash, cooked and mashed
3   tablespoons extra virgin olive oil

Makes 8 servings.
Each serving counts as 1 starchy vegetable, 1 vegetable, and 1 fat.

Nutrition Facts

Calories 150	Calories from Fat 45

% Daily Value*

Total Fat 5g	**8%**
Saturated Fat 1g	**5%**
Trans Fat 0g	
Cholesterol 0mg	**0%**
Sodium 10mg	**0%**
Total Carbohydrate 25g	**8%**
Dietary Fiber 6g	**24%**
Sugars 8g	
Protein 3g	

Vitamin A 230%	•	Vitamin C 45%
Calcium 8%	•	Iron 6%

*Percent Daily Values are based on a 2,000 calorie diet. Your daily values may be higher or lower depending on your calorie needs:

		Calories:	2,000	2,500
Total Fat	Less than		65g	80g
Saturated Fat	Less than		20g	25g
Cholesterol	Less than		300mg	300mg
Sodium	Less than		2,400mg	2,400mg
Total Carbohydrate			300g	375g
Dietary Fiber			25g	30g

Calories per gram:
Fat 9 • Carbohydrate 4 • Protein 4

Sweet and Sour Red Cabbage

1 medium red onion, cut in half
  and finely sliced
1–2 tablespoons olive oil
1 medium head red cabbage,
  finely shredded (core removed)
1 medium Granny Smith apple,
  coarsely chopped
½ cup red wine vinegar
  (or ¼ cup red wine and
  ¼ cup red wine vinegar)
1 tablespoon light brown sugar
  Salt and pepper to taste
  (optional)

**Makes 8 (½-cup) servings.
Each serving counts as 2
vegetables and 1 fat.**

Our version of this Austrian and German favorite uses apple and onion in place of some of the sugar and the bacon. It is traditional with meats usually served at Christmas. The cabbage provides vivid color on the winter table as well as plenty of antioxidants. Make it ahead because it tastes even better the following day. And any leftovers make a great side dish with lunch or as a snack all by itself.

Heat olive oil in a large skillet over medium heat.

Sauté onions until translucent (3–5 minutes).

Add the shredded cabbage and cook for another 5 minutes until it starts to wilt. Add the apple, vinegar, and sugar and decrease the heat to low. Cover and cook for another 30 minutes or so (and up to 2–3 hours), stirring occasionally.

Season with salt and pepper if desired.

Nutrition Facts

Calories 90	Calories from Fat 30

% Daily Value*

Total Fat 3.5g	**5%**
Saturated Fat 0.5g	**3%**
Trans Fat 0g	
Cholesterol 0mg	**0%**
Sodium 30mg	**1%**
Total Carbohydrate 14g	**5%**
Dietary Fiber 3g	**12%**
Sugars 9g	
Protein 2g	

Vitamin A 25%	•	Vitamin C 100%
Calcium 6%	•	Iron 6%

*Percent Daily Values are based on a 2,000 calorie diet. Your daily values may be higher or lower depending on your calorie needs:

		Calories:	2,000	2,500
Total Fat	Less than		65g	80g
Saturated Fat	Less than		20g	25g
Cholesterol	Less than		300mg	300mg
Sodium	Less than		2,400mg	2,400mg
Total Carbohydrate			300g	375g
Dietary Fiber			25g	30g

Calories per gram:
Fat 9 • Carbohydrate 4 • Protein 4

Tomato and Fennel Bisque

● ● ● ● ● ● ● ● ● ● ● ● ● ● ● ● ●

This is the next best thing to a fresh tomato soup, packed with flavor and nutrients, and none of the starch added to canned tomato soup. And you can reduce the sodium significantly by using unsalted canned tomato chunks or by using fresh tomatoes if you have them. This is probably my favorite soup any time of year

●

In a large saucepan or small stockpot, heat 2 tablespoons olive oil. Add the chopped vegetables and sauté for 15 minutes over medium heat until they are soft and golden brown.

Add the tomatoes, broth, and thyme and continue to cook for another 10 minutes or until the fennel is tender.

Using a handheld immersion blender, puree the soup but leave some texture to the mixture.

Add the milk and heat for another minute or so.

Garnish with a tablespoon of low-fat crumbled feta cheese and chopped fennel fronds.

2 tablespoons olive oil
1 medium onion, chopped coarsely
4 large garlic cloves, chopped coarsely
1 large fennel bulb (about 1 pound), chopped coarsely (½- to 1-inch dice)
1 (16-ounce) can light chicken broth (or 2 cups homemade chicken broth)
2 (16–ounce) cans fire-roasted tomato chunks or 2½ pound of fresh plum or other tomatoes (cut in half, squeeze to remove the seeds)
1 teaspoon dried leaf thyme or 1 tablespoon fresh chopped thyme
1 cup nonfat milk
Season with salt and pepper (optional)
4 tablespoons crumbled low-fat feta cheese for garnish

Makes 8 (1-cup) servings.
Each serving counts as 3 vegetables and 1 fat.

Nutrition Facts

Calories 110 — Calories from Fat 35

% Daily Value*

	% Daily Value*
Total Fat 4g	**6%**
Saturated Fat 1g	**5%**
Trans Fat 0g	
Cholesterol 0mg	**0%**
Sodium 520mg	**22%**
Total Carbohydrate 16g	**5%**
Dietary Fiber 3g	**12%**
Sugars 9g	
Protein 5g	

Vitamin A 25% • Vitamin C 40%
Calcium 6% • Iron 6%

*Percent Daily Values are based on a 2,000 calorie diet. Your daily values may be higher or lower depending on your calorie needs:

		Calories:	2,000	2,500
Total Fat	Less than		65g	80g
Saturated Fat	Less than		20g	25g
Cholesterol	Less than		300mg	300mg
Sodium	Less than		2,400mg	2,400mg
Total Carbohydrate			300g	375g
Dietary Fiber			25g	30g

Calories per gram:
Fat 9 • Carbohydrate 4 • Protein 4

Tomato Harvest Salad

. . . .

1   **pound red tomatoes**
½   **pound cherry or**
     pear tomatoes, any color
½   **pound yellow or**
     orange tomatoes
1   **medium red onion,**
     halved and sliced thinly
2   **tablespoons olive oil**
4–6 **small cloves garlic, sliced thinly**
⅓   **cup basil leaves torn into pieces**
3   **sprigs basil for garnish**
     Black pepper to taste
½   **teaspoon salt (optional)**

Makes 6 servings.
Each serving counts as 2
vegetables and 1 fat.

This salad is best when fresh tomatoes are harvested in late summer and early fall from your garden or found at a farmers' market. I always plant at least three colors of tomatoes just to prepare this salad often during harvest season and also to enjoy the color of the tomatoes on the vine.

Cut the tomatoes into approximately 2-inch chunks, leaving the smallest tomatoes whole, quartering the medium tomatoes, and cutting the larger ones into eighths. Place in a large bowl and toss with red onions and black pepper. Add salt if desired.

Sauté the garlic slices in olive oil over low heat, cooking and turning occasionally for 5–10 minutes or until the garlic is a light golden color. Pour the oil and garlic into a small dish to cool to room temperature.

Just before serving, place the tomato mixture into a serving bowl or on a platter. Dress the salad with the garlic slices, oil, and torn basil leaves. Garnish with sprigs of whole basil.

Serve at room temperature for best flavor. This is one recipe that is unlikely to have leftovers.

Nutrition Facts

Calories 90   Calories from Fat 45

% Daily Value*

Total Fat 5g	**8%**
Saturated Fat 0.5g	**3%**
Trans Fat 0g	
Cholesterol 0mg	**0%**
Sodium 5mg	**0%**
Total Carbohydrate 10g	**3%**
Dietary Fiber 1g	**4%**
Sugars 5g	
Protein 1g	

Vitamin A 4%	•	Vitamin C 45%
Calcium 4%	•	Iron 2%

*Percent Daily Values are based on a 2,000 calorie diet. Your daily values may be higher or lower depending on your calorie needs:

		Calories:	2,000	2,500
Total Fat	Less than		65g	80g
Saturated Fat	Less than		20g	25g
Cholesterol	Less than		300mg	300mg
Sodium	Less than		2,400mg	2,400mg
Total Carbohydrate			300g	375g
Dietary Fiber			25g	30g

Calories per gram:
    Fat 9 • Carbohydrate 4 • Protein 4

Vegetable Potpourri

This recipe is an adaptation of the Romanian Vegetable Potpourri that appeared in the original 3D book *Your Whole Life*. It's a great dish any time of year, and the vegetables can be varied depending on what's available and what's in season at the market or in your garden.

In a Dutch oven or large pot, sauté onions over medium heat for 5 minutes. Add the garlic and cook for another 1–2 minutes.

Add the remaining vegetables, broth, and seasonings and bring to a boil. Lower the heat, cover the pot, and simmer, stirring occasionally, for 20–25 minutes or until the liquid is absorbed and the vegetables are tender. Add more broth and continue cooking if necessary.

2 medium Vidalia onions, cut into wedges
4 garlic cloves, crushed
1–2 tablespoons extra virgin olive oil
1 medium eggplant, ½-inch dice
2 medium tomatoes, peeled and coarsely chopped, or 1 cup unsalted diced canned tomatoes
1 bell pepper (any color), 1-inch dice
1 small summer squash or zucchini, 1-inch dice
1 medium potato (6 ounces), ½-inch dice
1 cup light or homemade chicken broth
¼ teaspoon fresh ground black pepper

Makes 6 (½-cup) servings.
Each serving counts as 2 vegetables and 1 fat.

Nutrition Facts

Calories 90 Calories from Fat 40

	% Daily Value*
Total Fat 5g	8%
Saturated Fat 0.5g	3%
Trans Fat 0g	
Cholesterol 0mg	0%
Sodium 140mg	6%
Total Carbohydrate 11g	4%
Dietary Fiber 2g	8%
Sugars 3g	
Protein 3g	

Vitamin A 2%	•	Vitamin C 30%	
Calcium 4%	•	Iron 4%	

*Percent Daily Values are based on a 2,000 calorie diet. Your daily values may be higher or lower depending on your calorie needs:

		Calories:	2,000	2,500
Total Fat	Less than		65g	80g
Saturated Fat	Less than		20g	25g
Cholesterol	Less than		300mg	300mg
Sodium	Less than		2,400mg	2,400mg
Total Carbohydrate			300g	375g
Dietary Fiber			25g	30g

Calories per gram:
Fat 9 • Carbohydrate 4 • Protein 4

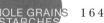

Anadama Batter Bread

. . . .

If you haven't made homemade bread before, this is an easy way to try your hand at it. And even if you're an experienced baker, you'll love the difference of this loaf.

¾ cup boiling water
½ cup whole-grain cornmeal
3 tablespoons light olive oil
¼ cup molasses
1 teaspoon salt
1 package of active dry yeast
¼ cup warm water
    (approx. 110 degrees — check
    with a thermometer)
1 large egg
1 cup whole-wheat flour
1¾ cup white whole-wheat flour

Makes 12 thick slices or 24 thin slices. Each thick slice counts as 2 whole grains and 1 fat.

Spray a 9 x 5 x 3-inch metal loaf pan with nonstick spray.

Place the cornmeal in a medium bowl. Pour the boiling water over it and add the oil, molasses, and salt. Mix to combine and let cool to lukewarm.

In the bowl of your standing mixer, pour the warm water and sprinkle the envelope of yeast over it. Stir to dissolve.

Add the cornmeal mixture to the yeast and water. Add the egg and 1 cup of the white whole-wheat flour. Turn the mixer to medium speed and beat for 1 minute. Add 1 cup of the whole-wheat flour and mix for another minute. Add the remaining ¾ cup of flour and beat for another minute. (You can also use a food processor if you don't have a stand mixer.)

Pour the batter into the prepared loaf pan and tap the pan on the counter to level the batter. Cover with waxed paper and a towel and put it in a warm place to rise, away from drafts and cold countertops, for approximately 1 1/2 hours or as long as it takes to double the size of the batter in the pan.

Preheat the oven to 375 degrees.

Sprinkle the top of the loaf with 1–2 teaspoons additional cornmeal and kosher salt if desired.

Bake the loaf for about 50–60 minutes or until it sounds hollow when rapped with your knuckle. Turn out onto a cooling rack.

Nutrition Facts

Calories 190	Calories from Fat 40	
		% Daily Value*
Total Fat 5g		**8%**
Saturated Fat 0.5g		**3%**
Trans Fat 0g		
Cholesterol 20mg		**7%**
Sodium 200mg		**8%**
Total Carbohydrate 32g		**11%**
Dietary Fiber 4g		**16%**
Sugars 4g		
Protein 5g.		
Vitamin A 0%	• Vitamin C 0%	
Calcium 2%	• Iron 10%	

*Percent Daily Values are based on a 2,000 calorie diet. Your daily values may be higher or lower depending on your calorie needs:

		Calories:	2,000	2,500
Total Fat	Less than		65g	80g
Saturated Fat	Less than		20g	25g
Cholesterol	Less than		300mg	300mg
Sodium	Less than		2,400mg	2,400mg
Total Carbohydrate			300g	375g
Dietary Fiber			25g	30g

Calories per gram:
    Fat 9 • Carbohydrate 4 • Protein 4

Baked Barley Mushroom Risotto

• •

Barley is an excellent source of water-soluble fiber, which is also found in oatmeal. This is a simple side dish that is inexpensive, delicious, and good for your heart. I like to cook this in a heavy 2-quart casserole that has a tight-fitting lid so the moisture stays in the pan while cooking. Spray the casserole interior with nonstick spray so that you can easily spoon every morsel of the risotto after it's cooked.

•

Preheat the oven to 350 degrees.

In a skillet sauté chopped onion in olive oil over medium heat for about 3–5 minutes. Add the mushrooms and cook for another 4 minutes, stirring occasionally. Add the barley and continue cooking for another 2 minutes.

Season with salt and pepper if desired, then pour the mixture into a 2-quart casserole. Pour boiling water over the ingredients to cover them plus another ½ inch.

Cover tightly and bake for 20–30 minutes or until the barley is tender. Check after 15 minutes to see if you need to add more liquid for the barley to cook thoroughly. Add only ¼ cup water or broth at a time, and return casserole to the oven for an additional 5 minutes or until the barley is tender.

Garnish with parsley and Parmesan.

1 large onion, chopped fine
3 tablespoons olive oil
1 8-ounce package of sliced button or baby bella mushrooms
1 cup pearl barley
2 16–ounce) cans low-sodium beef broth
Salt and pepper to taste (optional)
3 tablespoons chopped fresh parsley
1 tablespoon grated Parmesan cheese

Makes 9 (½-cup) servings.
Each serving counts as 1 whole grain, 1 vegetable, and 1 fat.

Nutrition Facts		
Calories 150	Calories from Fat 50	
		% Daily Value*
Total Fat 6g		9%
Saturated Fat 1g		5%
Trans Fat 0g		
Cholesterol 0mg		0%
Sodium 45mg		2%
Total Carbohydrate 20g		7%
Dietary Fiber 4g		16%
Sugars 2g		
Protein 5g		
Vitamin A 2%	•	Vitamin C 4%
Calcium 4%	•	Iron 6%

*Percent Daily Values are based on a 2,000 calorie diet. Your daily values may be higher or lower depending on your calorie needs:

		Calories:	2,000	2,500
Total Fat	Less than		65g	80g
Saturated Fat	Less than		20g	25g
Cholesterol	Less than		300mg	300mg
Sodium	Less than		2,400mg	2,400mg
Total Carbohydrate			300g	375g
Dietary Fiber			25g	30g

Calories per gram:
Fat 9 • Carbohydrate 4 • Protein 4

Corny Southwestern Cornbread

2 cups yellow whole-grain medium-grind cornmeal (such as Bob's Red Mill)
2 tablespoons sugar
1½ teaspoons baking powder
1 teaspoon salt
2 eggs, beaten lightly
⅔ cup nonfat milk
¼ cup light olive oil or grape seed oil
1 cup (8-ounce can) creamed corn
½ cup (4-ounce can) mild green chilies, diced

Makes 18 servings.
Each serving counts as 1 whole grain and 1 fat.

This cornbread is truly whole-grain because it's made with 100 percent corn and no flour. Creamed corn makes it moist and adds another layer of corn flavor. You can leave out the chili peppers if you prefer a milder flavor. Or you can add ¼ cup chopped herbs such as dill, basil, or parsley.

Set the oven to 400 degrees. Spray an 8-inch square baking pan with nonstick cooking spray.

In a medium bowl combine the dry ingredients.

In a small bowl combine the rest of the ingredients. Add to the dry ingredients and mix very lightly until just combined.

Pour into baking pan and bake for 18–25 minutes or just until top begins to brown. Cool on a baking rack for 10 minutes before cutting into 9 squares. Then cut each square in half to a rectangle.

Nutrition Facts

Calories 110   Calories from Fat 40

	% Daily Value*
Total Fat 4.5g	7%
Saturated Fat 0g	0%
Trans Fat 0g	
Cholesterol 25mg	8%
Sodium 240mg	10%
Total Carbohydrate 15g	5%
Dietary Fiber 3g	12%
Sugars 3g	
Protein 2g	

Vitamin A 2%	•	Vitamin C 2%
Calcium 2%	•	Iron 4%

*Percent Daily Values are based on a 2,000 calorie diet. Your daily values may be higher or lower depending on your calorie needs:

		Calories:	2,000	2,500
Total Fat	Less than		65g	80g
Saturated Fat	Less than		20g	25g
Cholesterol	Less than		300mg	300mg
Sodium	Less than		2,400mg	2,400mg
Total Carbohydrate			300g	375g
Dietary Fiber			25g	30g

Calories per gram:
Fat 9 • Carbohydrate 4 • Protein 4

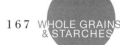

Dijon Potato Salad

This potato salad is creamy but very low in fat. It is easy to make for a crowd by doubling or tripling the recipe. Garnish with freshly picked, cooked green beans and chunks of light tuna to make a meal with a distinct French touch.

Add all of the ingredients except the potatoes to a large bowl. Whisk to blend thoroughly.

Add the potatoes and toss until coated. Chill for at least 1 hour before serving.

1 pound small red bliss potatoes, cooked and cut into quarters or ¾-inch chunks
½ cup nonfat plain Greek yogurt
¼ cup low-fat mayonnaise
1 tablespoon Dijon mustard
1 teaspoon whole mustard seeds
1 teaspoon cider vinegar
½ teaspoon fresh ground white pepper
2 tablespoons fresh chopped tarragon or 1 bunch scallions, sliced thinly

Makes 6 servings.
Each serving counts as 1 starch and 1 vegetable.

Nutrition Facts

Calories 90   Calories from Fat 10

	% Daily Value*
Total Fat 1.5g	2%
Saturated Fat 0g	0%
Trans Fat 0g	
Cholesterol 0mg	0%
Sodium 150mg	6%
Total Carbohydrate 16g	5%
Dietary Fiber 1g	4%
Sugars 1g	
Protein 3g	

Vitamin A 0%   •   Vitamin C 25%
Calcium 2%   •   Iron 4%

*Percent Daily Values are based on a 2,000 calorie diet. Your daily values may be higher or lower depending on your calorie needs:

		Calories:	2,000	2,500
Total Fat	Less than		65g	80g
Saturated Fat	Less than		20g	25g
Cholesterol	Less than		300mg	300mg
Sodium	Less than		2,400mg	2,400mg
Total Carbohydrate			300g	375g
Dietary Fiber			25g	30g

Calories per gram:
Fat 9 • Carbohydrate 4 • Protein 4

Green Rice

● ● ● ● ● ● ● ● ● ● ● ● ● ● ● ● ● ● ● ●

1½ cups brown basmati rice
2   tablespoons olive oil
1   medium onion,
    coarsely chopped
1   small bunch flat-leaf parsley,
    chopped (about 1½ cups)
1   bunch cilantro, chopped
    (about 1 cup)
1   cup fresh dill or baby spinach,
    chopped
3   cups water or homemade
    chicken broth
1   tablespoon chopped garlic
1   teaspoon turmeric
    Salt and pepper to taste
    (optional)

Try this whole-grain rice dish packed with antioxidants, vitamins, and minerals. If you don't have fresh herbs on hand, you can use a small bag of baby spinach and chop it before adding to the rice.

●

Heat oil in a large saucepan over medium heat. Add the chopped onion and cook until translucent but not brown. Add the rice and continue to cook for another 3–5 minutes.

Add all of the chopped herbs, garlic, and turmeric to the rice and combine completely. Add the water or chicken broth and bring to a boil. Stir once. Cover and reduce the heat to a simmer and cook for approximately 45 minutes. Check for doneness, adding additional water and time if necessary.

Remove from heat and let stand for another 10 minutes in the covered pot. Fluff with a fork before serving.

Makes 12 (½-cup) servings. Each serving counts as 1 whole grain and 1 vegetable.

Nutrition Facts

Calories 110   Calories from Fat 20

% Daily Value*

	% Daily Value*
Total Fat 2g	3%
Saturated Fat 0g	0%
Trans Fat 0g	
Cholesterol 0mg	0%
Sodium 5mg	0%
Total Carbohydrate 20g	7%
Dietary Fiber 1g	4%
Sugars 1g	
Protein 2g	

Vitamin A 15%   •   Vitamin C 20%
Calcium 2%   •   Iron 6%

*Percent Daily Values are based on a 2,000 calorie diet. Your daily values may be higher or lower depending on your calorie needs:

		Calories:	2,000	2,500
Total Fat	Less than		65g	80g
Saturated Fat	Less than		20g	25g
Cholesterol	Less than		300mg	300mg
Sodium	Less than		2,400mg	2,400mg
Total Carbohydrate			300g	375g
Dietary Fiber			25g	30g

Calories per gram:
Fat 9 • Carbohydrate 4 • Protein 4

Whole Grain and Bean Salad

A delicious way to combine whole grains, beans, and vegetables, this salad is a great example of how you can make whole, healthy foods quickly and inexpensively. You can make this with whole-wheat bulgur, cucumbers, and parsley for a tasty tabouleh or with quinoa, scallions, and cilantro for a Southwestern variation.

Combine all ingredients and toss. Let stand for 30 minutes before serving to allow the flavors to blend.

Serve at room temperature as an entrée on a bed of greens, or serve hot as a side dish. Leftovers can be added to a salad for tomorrow's lunch.

1   can black beans, rinsed and drained
1½ cups cooked brown rice (such as Lundberg rice), bulgur, or quinoa
1   small red onion or 1 bunch scallions, chopped coarsely
2   plum tomatoes, chopped
1   red, green, or yellow pepper, chopped (or 1 cup chopped cucumber)
½   jalapeño pepper, seeded and chopped (optional)
2   tablespoons lime juice
2   tablespoons olive oil
¼   cup chopped parsley or cilantro
    Salt and pepper to taste (optional)

Makes 8 servings.
Each serving counts as 1 vegetable, 1 whole grain, and 1 fat.

Nutrition Facts

Calories 120	Calories from Fat 40	
		% Daily Value*
Total Fat 4.5g		7%
Saturated Fat 0.5g		3%
Trans Fat 0g		
Cholesterol 0mg		0%
Sodium 210mg		9%
Total Carbohydrate 18g		6%
Dietary Fiber 4g		16%
Sugars 2g		
Protein 5g		
Vitamin A 4%	•	Vitamin C 35%
Calcium 2%	•	Iron 8%

*Percent Daily Values are based on a 2,000 calorie diet. Your daily values may be higher or lower depending on your calorie needs:

		Calories:	2,000	2,500
Total Fat	Less than		65g	80g
Saturated Fat	Less than		20g	25g
Cholesterol	Less than		300mg	300mg
Sodium	Less than		2,400mg	2,400mg
Total Carbohydrate			300g	375g
Dietary Fiber			25g	30g

Calories per gram:
Fat 9 • Carbohydrate 4 • Protein 4

Cannoli Cream

1 cup low-fat ricotta cheese
3 tablespoons all-fruit orange
   marmalade
¼ teaspoon vanilla extract
⅛ teaspoon orange extract
1 tablespoon chopped pistachios
1 ounce coarsely chopped dark
   chocolate

Makes 6 servings.
Each serving counts as 1 fat, ½
starch, and ½ protein.

I have always loved the taste of Italian cannoli pastries, and this version captures the creamy flavor with many fewer calories. It's especially good served with fresh berries when they're at their peak in summer. I once served this as a parfait in champagne glasses layered with blackberries and raspberries for a July Fourth party.

In a small food processor or standing mixer, whip the ricotta until it's really smooth. Scrape down the bowl as necessary. Add a few drops of milk if required to achieve the consistency of thick whipped cream.

Add the marmalade and pulse briefly so that chunks of the orange remain identifiable.

Put the mixture into a small bowl and stir in the extracts. Add the nuts and chocolate and fold in gently until mixed. Chill until serving.

Nutrition Facts

Calories 100	Calories from Fat 45	
		% Daily Value*
Total Fat 5g		8%
Saturated Fat 3g		15%
Trans Fat 0g		
Cholesterol 15mg		5%
Sodium 65mg		3%
Total Carbohydrate 10g		3%
Dietary Fiber 1g		4%
Sugars 8g		
Protein 4g		
Vitamin A 2%	•	Vitamin C 0%
Calcium 6%	•	Iron 0%

*Percent Daily Values are based on a 2,000 calorie diet. Your daily values may be higher or lower depending on your calorie needs:

		Calories:	2,000	2,500
Total Fat	Less than		65g	80g
Saturated Fat	Less than		20g	25g
Cholesterol	Less than		300mg	300mg
Sodium	Less than		2,400mg	2,400mg
Total Carbohydrate			300g	375g
Dietary Fiber			25g	30g

Calories per gram:
Fat 9 • Carbohydrate 4 • Protein 4

Fruit Crisp

Crisps can be a delicious dessert, made with any fruit that is in season. They taste great and help satisfy your need for fruit and for whole-grain ingredients, but they are less sweet and lower in calories than a cake or a pie. You can use any single fruit or combine fruits such as peaches and pears or nectarines and raspberries.

Preheat the oven to 375 degrees.

Spray a 9-inch pie pan or an 8-inch square baking pan with a nonstick spray.

Peel, core, and cut the fruit into ¾-inch chunks and place in the prepared baking pan. Sprinkle with lemon juice and grated lemon rind and toss to coat.

Combine the rest of the ingredients except the walnuts in a food processor just until the mixture is chunky. Add the walnuts and pulse 3 times.

Pour the crumb mixture onto the fruit and bake for 20–25 minutes or until the fruit is fork-tender and the topping is lightly browned.

4 peaches, nectarines, apples, or pears (total of 2 pounds of fruit)
2 tablespoons lemon juice
Grated rind of 1 lemon
1 tablespoon butter
1 tablespoon walnut oil (or canola oil)
1 tablespoon brown sugar
¼ cup whole-wheat pastry flour
½ cup old-fashioned oats (not quick or instant)
1 teaspoon cinnamon or cardamom
¼ cup walnuts, coarsely chopped

Makes 4 servings.
Each serving counts as 1 fruit, ½ whole grain, and 1 fat.

Nutrition Facts

Calories 150   Calories from Fat 50

	% Daily Value*
Total Fat 6g	9%
Saturated Fat 1.5g	8%
Trans Fat 0g	
Cholesterol 5mg	2%
Sodium 15mg	1%
Total Carbohydrate 26g	9%
Dietary Fiber 5g	20%
Sugars 13g	
Protein 2g	

Vitamin A 2% • Vitamin C 10%
Calcium 2% • Iron 4%

*Percent Daily Values are based on a 2,000 calorie diet. Your daily values may be higher or lower depending on your calorie needs:

	Calories:	2,000	2,500
Total Fat	Less than	65g	80g
Saturated Fat	Less than	20g	25g
Cholesterol	Less than	300mg	300mg
Sodium	Less than	2,400mg	2,400mg
Total Carbohydrate		300g	375g
Dietary Fiber		25g	30g

Calories per gram:
Fat 9 • Carbohydrate 4 • Protein 4

Golden Oldie
Oatmeal Raisin Cookies

● ● ● ● ● ● ● ● ● ● ● ● ● ● ● ● ● ● ● ●

2 sticks of butter,
  at room temperature
¾ cup packed light brown sugar
¾ cup granulated white sugar
2 large eggs
1 cup unbleached white flour
½ cup whole-wheat flour
1 teaspoon salt
1½ teaspoons baking powder
1 teaspoon fresh grated nutmeg
3 cups old-fashioned rolled oats
1½ cups golden raisins

Makes 48 (1-ounce) cookies.
Each cookie counts as 1 whole
grain and 1 fat.

These are similar to the classic oatmeal cookies I grew up
with. Sometimes you just can't improve on a good thing. I
recommend using fresh ground nutmeg to boost the flavor
significantly. You don't have to buy a special grater for the
nutmeg—just use a rasp or a stand-type cheese grater.

●

Preheat oven to 350 degrees. Cut parchment paper to fit your
baking sheets.

Using an electric mixer, beat the butter until it's creamy and
lighter in color. Add both sugars and beat until light and fluffy,
3–5 minutes. Beat in each egg separately, for another minute
after each one is added.

Measure the flours, salt, baking powder, and nutmeg onto
a sheet of wax paper. Mix together to distribute ingredients
evenly. Add to the mixer bowl and blend into the butter mixture
on low speed. Then add the oatmeal and raisins, mixing in
gently on the lowest speed. Remove bowl from the mixer. Use
a large rubber spatula to scrape down the sides and finish
folding in the oats and raisins.

Using a 1-ounce ice cream scoop, form rounded scoops and
place on parchment-lined baking sheets. Bake for 13–15
minutes, checking after 10 minutes. Rotate the baking sheets
if one edge starts to turn brown too quickly. The cookies are
done when the edges start to turn golden brown. Cool the pan
on a cooling rack for 30 minutes. Store in airtight containers
when completely cool. Cookies will keep for 7 days at room
temperature or 1–2 months in the freezer. You can even
scoop out the dough, place on baking sheets, and freeze.
Then place in a zipper-type plastic bag in your freezer—bake
a few at a time when you want them.

Nutrition Facts

Calories 110   Calories from Fat 40

% Daily Value*

	% Daily Value*
Total Fat 4.5g	**7%**
Saturated Fat 2.5g	**13%**
Trans Fat 0g	
Cholesterol 20mg	**7%**
Sodium 80mg	**3%**
Total Carbohydrate 16g	**5%**
Dietary Fiber 1g	**4%**
Sugars 9g	
Protein 2g	

Vitamin A 2% • Vitamin C 0%

Calcium 2% • Iron 2%

*Percent Daily Values are based on a 2,000 calorie diet. Your daily values may be higher or lower depending on your calorie needs:

		Calories:	2,000	2,500
Total Fat	Less than		65g	80g
Saturated Fat	Less than		20g	25g
Cholesterol	Less than		300mg	300mg
Sodium	Less than		2,400mg	2,400mg
Total Carbohydrate			300g	375g
Dietary Fiber			25g	30g

Calories per gram:
Fat 9 • Carbohydrate 4 • Protein 4

Maple-baked Apples

Baked apples are a classic dessert or can even be served as a accompaniment to a pork roast or chop. They are easy to prepare and provide just enough sweetness with a minimum of added sugar.

Preheat the oven to 350 degrees.

Core the apples. Peel the top half of each apple and place them in a baking dish or pie pan.

Mix the brown sugar and spices together. Sprinkle over the apples and into the cores.

Drizzle the maple syrup over the apples and into the cores.

Add the maple extract and water to the cider and pour it into the baking dish around the apples.

Cover the apples with aluminum foil and bake for 10 minutes, then baste with the cider; repeat this step every 10 minutes (40–50 minutes total) or until the apples are fork-tender.

Remove from the oven and cool for 15–30 minutes before serving. Reheat leftovers in the microwave for 15–20 seconds before serving.

4   cooking apples,
    such as Cortland or Golden
    Delicious (total of 2 pounds)

1   tablespoon light brown sugar

¼   teaspoon cinnamon

⅛   teaspoon freshly ground
    nutmeg

2   tablespoons maple syrup

1   teaspoon maple extract

½   cup apple cider or
    unsweetened apple juice

½   cup water

**Makes 4 servings
(including fruit and sauce).
Each serving counts as 1 fruit
and 1 starch.**

To save another 25 Calories, serve with a slotted spoon or spatula, leaving the liquid in the pan.

Nutrition Facts			
Calories 170	Calories from Fat 5		
	% Daily Value*		
Total Fat 0g	0%		
Saturated Fat 0g	0%		
Trans Fat 0g			
Cholesterol 0mg	0%		
Sodium 5mg	0%		
Total Carbohydrate 44g	15%		
Dietary Fiber 5g	20%		
Sugars 35g			
Protein 1g			
Vitamin A 2%	• Vitamin C 15%		
Calcium 2%	• Iron 2%		

*Percent Daily Values are based on a 2,000 calorie diet. Your daily values may be higher or lower depending on your calorie needs:

		Calories:	2,000	2,500
Total Fat	Less than		65g	80g
Saturated Fat	Less than		20g	25g
Cholesterol	Less than		300mg	300mg
Sodium	Less than		2,400mg	2,400mg
Total Carbohydrate			300g	375g
Dietary Fiber			25g	30g

Calories per gram:
Fat 9 • Carbohydrate 4 • Protein 4

Peach, Blueberry, and Lime Compote

3 medium, ripe peaches, peeled and cut into 8 wedges each
½ pint blueberries
   Zest and juice of 1 lime
2 teaspoons confectioners or superfine sugar

Makes 4 servings.
Each serving counts as 1 fruit.

Fresh fruit in season is wonderful all by itself, but when you want to offer a more elegant fresh fruit dessert, this is perfect. Serve in a beautiful goblet or in an ordinary custard cup and enjoy the juicy sweet and tart flavors of this combination.

Combine all ingredients and toss. Let stand for 30 minutes before serving to allow the flavors to blend.

Serve at room temperature or chilled.

Nutrition Facts			
Calories 70	Calories from Fat 5		
	% Daily Value*		
Total Fat 0g	0%		
Saturated Fat 0g	0%		
Trans Fat 0g			
Cholesterol 0mg	0%		
Sodium 0mg	0%		
Total Carbohydrate 18g	6%		
Dietary Fiber 3g	12%		
Sugars 14g			
Protein 1g			
Vitamin A 8%	• Vitamin C 20%		
Calcium 0%	• Iron 2%		

*Percent Daily Values are based on a 2,000 calorie diet. Your daily values may be higher or lower depending on your calorie needs:

		Calories:	2,000	2,500
Total Fat	Less than		65g	80g
Saturated Fat	Less than		20g	25g
Cholesterol	Less than		300mg	300mg
Sodium	Less than		2,400mg	2,400mg
Total Carbohydrate			300g	375g
Dietary Fiber			25g	30g

Calories per gram:
Fat 9 • Carbohydrate 4 • Protein 4

Pumpkin Pie Pudding

Traditional pumpkin pie with the crust has two to three times the calories of this fall favorite. It's a great light ending to a richer than usual holiday meal. And how often can you count a dessert as a serving of vegetable?

Preheat oven to 325 degrees.

Prepare 8 (6-ounce) custard cups or ramekins by spraying with nonstick spray. Place them in a baking pan or roasting pan.

Place pumpkin and egg whites in a large bowl and whisk together well. Add the sugar and spices to the bowl and whisk again until they are combined. Then add the evaporated milk and blend until smooth.

Divide the mixture among the cups or ramekins. Fill the pan with hot water to 1 inch below the ramekins and place in the oven to bake for approximately 30–40 minutes or until the pudding has set. The time will vary depending on the size of the baking dishes.

1 can (16-ounce) pureed pumpkin or 2 cups cooked and mashed fresh pumpkin
4 egg whites
½ cup light brown sugar, packed
1 teaspoon ground cinnamon
½ teaspoon ground ginger
¼ teaspoon freshly grated nutmeg
¼ teaspoon ground cloves
1 (12-ounce) can fat-free evaporated milk
Optional garnish (2 tablespoons light aerosol whipped cream)

Makes 8 servings.
Each serving counts as 1 vegetable, 1 starch, and ½ lean protein.

Nutrition Facts

Calories 120   Calories from Fat 0

	% Daily Value*
Total Fat 0g	0%
Saturated Fat 0g	0%
Trans Fat 0g	
Cholesterol 0mg	0%
Sodium 95mg	4%
Total Carbohydrate 24g	8%
Dietary Fiber 2g	8%
Sugars 21g	
Protein 6g	

Vitamin A 170% • Vitamin C 0%
Calcium 15% • Iron 2%

*Percent Daily Values are based on a 2,000 calorie diet. Your daily values may be higher or lower depending on your calorie needs:

		Calories:	2,000	2,500
Total Fat	Less than		65g	80g
Saturated Fat	Less than		20g	25g
Cholesterol	Less than		300mg	300mg
Sodium	Less than		2,400mg	2,400mg
Total Carbohydrate			300g	375g
Dietary Fiber			25g	30g

Calories per gram:
Fat 9 • Carbohydrate 4 • Protein 4

Spiced Poached Fruit

- 8 large Bartlett pears, peeled, cored, and quartered
- 2 Golden Delicious apples, peeled, cored, and quartered
- 24 dried apricots
- ½ cup golden raisins
- 1 tablespoon fresh slivered lemon zest, or 1 teaspoon dried lemon peel
- ½ teaspoon ground allspice
- 1 cinnamon stick
- 4 whole cloves
- 1½ cups white dessert wine or white grape juice
- ½ cup sugar

Makes 24 (⅓-cup) servings. Each serving counts as 1½ fruits.

On a trip to the Isle of Capri, I enjoyed many wonderful meals but I tried not to sample too many of the sweets that Italy has to offer. One night after dinner, the waitress came to us not with a sample of sweets but with a large tray of poached fruit. We could point out which fruits we wanted and she would plate them and serve us. This recipe is as close as I have come to duplicating that beautiful dessert and savoring the memories of that trip.

Combine all of the ingredients in a large pan and bring to a boil over medium high heat. Lower the heat to a simmer and cook until the fruit is fork-tender (20–30 minutes depending on the ripeness of the fruit). Serve warm or chilled.

Nutrition Facts

Calories 100   Calories from Fat 0

% Daily Value*

Total Fat 0g	0%
Saturated Fat 0g	0%
Trans Fat 0g	
Cholesterol 0mg	0%
Sodium 0mg	0%
Total Carbohydrate 24g	8%
Dietary Fiber 3g	12%
Sugars 14g	
Protein 1g	

Vitamin A 8% • Vitamin C 8%
Calcium 2% • Iron 2%

*Percent Daily Values are based on a 2,000 calorie diet. Your daily values may be higher or lower depending on your calorie needs:

		Calories:	2,000	2,500
Total Fat	Less than		65g	80g
Saturated Fat	Less than		20g	25g
Cholesterol	Less than		300mg	300mg
Sodium	Less than		2,400mg	2,400mg
Total Carbohydrate			300g	375g
Dietary Fiber			25g	30g

Calories per gram:
Fat 9 • Carbohydrate 4 • Protein 4

Chimichurri

Every summer my garden produces an abundance of parsley and other herbs, so I started making my own chimichurri sauce. It is a traditional Argentine parsley-garlic sauce for grilled meats, but it can be used on fish, eggs, bread, and vegetables. I found that there are dozens of variations, just as with pesto. The basic formula includes chopped fresh herbs such as flat-leaf parsley, cilantro, thyme, and rosemary (doesn't this sound Mediterranean?), garlic, and either lemon juice or some type of vinegar to add some acidic bite. Unlike pesto, there are no nuts or cheese included, but the taste is rich and the herbs contribute plenty of vitamins as well. A little goes a long way!

1 bunch flat-leaf parsley (or ½ bunch each parsley and cilantro)
⅓ cup lemon juice, sherry vinegar, or red wine vinegar
8 cloves garlic, crushed (more if you like)
1–3 tablespoons fresh oregano, chopped (or 1–3 teaspoons dried)
½ teaspoon Cayenne pepper or ½ teaspoon dried red pepper flakes
½–¾ cup olive oil
Salt and pepper to taste (optional)

Add the first five ingredients to a blender or food processor, and process until smooth but not completely pureed. Whisk or pulse in olive oil and season to taste. Serve at room temperature. Refrigerate leftovers but bring to room temperature before using.

Makes 24 (2-tablespoon) servings. Each serving counts as 1 fat.

Nutrition Facts

Calories 60	Calories from Fat 50	
		% Daily Value*
Total Fat 6g		9%
Saturated Fat 1g		5%
Trans Fat 0g		
Cholesterol 0mg		0%
Sodium 0mg		0%
Total Carbohydrate 1g		0%
Dietary Fiber 0g		0%
Sugars 0g		
Protein 0g		
Vitamin A 8%	• Vitamin C 15%	
Calcium 2%	• Iron 2%	

*Percent Daily Values are based on a 2,000 calorie diet. Your daily values may be higher or lower depending on your calorie needs:

		Calories:	2,000	2,500
Total Fat	Less than		65g	80g
Saturated Fat	Less than		20g	25g
Cholesterol	Less than		300mg	300mg
Sodium	Less than		2,400mg	2,400mg
Total Carbohydrate			300g	375g
Dietary Fiber			25g	30g

Calories per gram:
Fat 9 • Carbohydrate 4 • Protein 4

Gremolata

½ cup chopped fresh flat-leaf parsley
4 large garlic cloves, minced
Grated zest of 1 lemon
Fresh ground black pepper
Salt (optional)

Makes approximately 4 servings. Although gremolata contains vitamins, minerals, and antioxidants from the parsley, garlic, and lemon, it only contains about ¼ serving of vegetable.

This condiment is traditionally sprinkled on veal in Italy, but it is also wonderful sprinkled on vegetables or fish. It adds a punch of flavor and some vitamins without adding many calories or much sodium. The flavor is reminiscent of pesto but does not contain the added fat of olive oil, pine nuts, or Parmesan cheese. It's quick, inexpensive, and very satisfying.

Combine all of the ingredients in a small bowl and toss to combine well. Store in a covered container for up to 3 days.

Nutrition Facts

Calories 10	Calories from Fat 0	
		% Daily Value*
Total Fat 0g		**0%**
Saturated Fat 0g		**0%**
Trans Fat 0g		
Cholesterol 0mg		**0%**
Sodium 5mg		**0%**
Total Carbohydrate 2g		**1%**
Dietary Fiber 1g		**4%**
Sugars 0g		
Protein 1g		

Vitamin A 15%	•	Vitamin C 25%
Calcium 2%	•	Iron 4%

*Percent Daily Values are based on a 2,000 calorie diet. Your daily values may be higher or lower depending on your calorie needs:

		Calories:	2,000	2,500
Total Fat	Less than		65g	80g
Saturated Fat	Less than		20g	25g
Cholesterol	Less than		300mg	300mg
Sodium	Less than		2,400mg	2,400mg
Total Carbohydrate			300g	375g
Dietary Fiber			25g	30g

Calories per gram:
Fat 9 • Carbohydrate 4 • Protein 4

Nuts about Red Pepper Dip

Packed with flavor and antioxidants, this recipe is a delicious way to incorporate vegetables and nuts into a dip. The slice of bread may seem like an odd ingredient for a dip but it serves as a thickener and binder for the other ingredients. Serve the dip with raw vegetables and toasted pita bread wedges, or use as a dressing for salad or a sauce for chicken or fish.

Toast the walnuts in a medium skillet for 5 minutes over medium heat until golden and fragrant. Cool the walnuts, place in a food processor, and pulse 5 times.

Heat the olive oil in the same skillet over medium heat. Add onions and garlic, and cook until translucent but not browned. Cool and add to the food processor.

Add the remaining ingredients and process until the walnuts are very finely chopped and no large chunks remain. Scrape down the sides of the bowl as often as necessary to incorporate all of the ingredients.

½ cup walnuts
3 tablespoons extra virgin olive oil
½ cup onion, coarsely chopped
4 large garlic cloves, coarsely chopped
1 jar (12-ounce) roasted red peppers packed in water (rinsed, drained, blotted dry) or 2 cups fresh roasted red peppers, skins removed
⅓ cup fresh basil leaves, coarsely chopped
1 slice of bread (crust removed) torn into 1-inch pieces
2 tablespoons fresh lemon juice

Makes 10 (2-tablespoon) servings.
Each serving counts as
1 vegetable and 1 fat.

Nutrition Facts

Calories 80	Calories from Fat 60

	% Daily Value*
Total Fat 6g	9%
Saturated Fat 0.5g	3%
Trans Fat 0g	
Cholesterol 0mg	0%
Sodium 100mg	4%
Total Carbohydrate 6g	2%
Dietary Fiber 2g	8%
Sugars 2g	
Protein 2g	

Vitamin A 8%	•	Vitamin C 15%
Calcium 2%	•	Iron 2%

*Percent Daily Values are based on a 2,000 calorie diet. Your daily values may be higher or lower depending on your calorie needs:

		Calories:	2,000	2,500
Total Fat	Less than		65g	80g
Saturated Fat	Less than		20g	25g
Cholesterol	Less than		300mg	300mg
Sodium	Less than		2,400mg	2,400mg
Total Carbohydrate			300g	375g
Dietary Fiber			25g	30g

Calories per gram:
Fat 9 • Carbohydrate 4 • Protein 4

Romesco Sauce

1 (16–ounce) can fire roasted diced tomatoes, drained
3 tablespoons paprika
1 tablespoon mild chili powder
10 large garlic cloves or 1 whole head of garlic
1 ounce blanched almonds, preferably Spanish almonds
1 ounce blanched hazelnuts
1 slice whole-wheat bread
2 tablespoons parsley
½ cup olive oil
1 tablespoon sherry vinegar, preferably Spanish
Salt and pepper (optional)

Makes 24 (1 rounded tablespoon) servings. Each serving counts as 1 fat and ½ vegetable.

I discovered this pepper sauce on my first trip to Spain, where it was served with shrimp. It is the type of sauce that is used like pesto, since a little goes a long way. I love it with fish but it can also be thinned by whisking in some water and used as a dressing on vegetables, potatoes, or salads. The color is gorgeous and the taste is complex.

Roast the garlic in the oven at 350 degrees for approximately 30 minutes or until just starting to soften, being careful to check to make sure they don't burn. When they are roasted, squeeze the cloves out of the skin and place them in a food processor.

Add the tomatoes, spices, nuts, bread, parsley, and half of the olive oil. Process until the mixture is very smooth. Then add the remaining oil and season with salt and pepper if desired. You may need to add a little water to thin it to the consistency of heavy cream.

This sauce will keep for a week in the refrigerator, or longer in the freezer. Be sure to let it sit at room temperature for at least 30 minutes before serving.

Nutrition Facts

Calories 70	Calories from Fat 60

	% Daily Value*
Total Fat 6g	9%
Saturated Fat 1g	5%
Trans Fat 0g	
Cholesterol 0mg	0%
Sodium 50mg	2%
Total Carbohydrate 3g	1%
Dietary Fiber 1g	4%
Sugars 1g	
Protein 1g	

Vitamin A 8% • Vitamin C 8%
Calcium 2% • Iron 2%

*Percent Daily Values are based on a 2,000 calorie diet. Your daily values may be higher or lower depending on your calorie needs:

		Calories:	2,000	2,500
Total Fat	Less than		65g	80g
Saturated Fat	Less than		20g	25g
Cholesterol	Less than		300mg	300mg
Sodium	Less than		2,400mg	2,400mg
Total Carbohydrate			300g	375g
Dietary Fiber			25g	30g

Calories per gram:
Fat 9 • Carbohydrate 4 • Protein 4

Two by Two Spiced Nuts

· ·

A great recipe to make ahead and portion into individual servings for a quick snack, anytime, anywhere. You can combine any three varieties of nuts that you have on hand. Although these nuts are high in fat, it's primarily monounsaturated fat. You can combine ½ portions of nuts with 2 tablespoons of dried fruit for a lower-fat treat.

·

Preheat oven to 225 degrees.

Whisk egg whites in a large bowl until foamy. Add first 7 ingredients to egg whites and whisk in. Add nuts and toss to coat thoroughly. If desired, sprinkle with sugar or Splenda® and stir.

Spread the nut mixture over two jelly-roll pans or rimmed baking sheets, being careful to keep in single layer. Bake at 225 degrees, turning every 15–20 minutes until nuts are thoroughly toasted but not too brown (approximately 70–80 minutes total). Cool completely before placing in a large airtight container or into individual serving containers.

2 teaspoons ground cinnamon
2 teaspoons ground ginger
2 teaspoons ground cumin
2 teaspoons Chinese five-spice powder
2 teaspoons salt (optional)
2 teaspoons chili powder (optional)
¼ teaspoon garlic powder
2 egg whites
2 cups whole blanched almonds
2 cups pecans
2 cups walnut halves or whole blanched hazelnuts
2 tablespoons sugar or Splenda® (optional)

Makes 24 (¼-cup) servings.
Each serving counts as 1 protein and 3 fats.

Nutrition Facts

Calories 190   Calories from Fat 160

	% Daily Value*
Total Fat 18g	28%
Saturated Fat 1.5g	8%
Trans Fat 0g	
Cholesterol 0mg	0%
Sodium 10mg	0%
Total Carbohydrate 6g	2%
Dietary Fiber 3g	12%
Sugars 1g	
Protein 5g	

Vitamin A 2% • Vitamin C 2%
Calcium 4% • Iron 8%

*Percent Daily Values are based on a 2,000 calorie diet. Your daily values may be higher or lower depending on your calorie needs:

		Calories:	2,000	2,500
Total Fat	Less than		65g	80g
Saturated Fat	Less than		20g	25g
Cholesterol	Less than		300mg	300mg
Sodium	Less than		2,400mg	2,400mg
Total Carbohydrate			300g	375g
Dietary Fiber			25g	30g

Calories per gram:
Fat 9 • Carbohydrate 4 • Protein 4

Resources

Sources for nutrient information
FOR RECIPES AND MENUS IN THIS BOOK

Corinne Netzer's Complete Book of Food Counts, by Corinne Netzer

Food Processor software, ESHA

NutriBase software, NutriBase

Magazine RECIPE RESOURCES

Clean Eating	www.CleanEating.com
Eating Well	www.EatingWell.com
Everyday Food	www.MarthaStewart.com/Everyday
Nutrition Action Newsletter	www.CSPI.org
Today's Diet and Nutrition	www.TodaysDietandNutrition.com
Vegetarian Times	www.VegetarianTimes.com

Recommended books
NUTRITION

Eating on the Run: Nutritious Eating—From Airline Meals to Microwave Zapping, by Evelyn Tribole

Nutrition at Your Fingertips, by Elisa Zied

What Color is Your Diet? by David Heber, MD, PhD, with Susan Bowerman, MS, RD

RECIPES

The Art of Simple Food, by Alice Waters

Betty Crocker's Diabetes Cookbook: Everyday Meals, Easy as 1-2-3, by Betty Crocker Editors

The Cook's Encyclopedia of Soups, by Debra Mayhew

Eating Well Serves Two, by Jim Romanoff

Fast Food My Way, by Jacques Pepin

Healthy Eating 1-2-3, by Rozanne Gold

How to Cook Everything: The Basics, by Mark Bittman

How to Pick a Peach: The Search for Flavor from Farm to Table, by Russ Parsons

James McNair's Salads, by James McNair and Jim Hildreth

Lickety Split Meals for Health Conscious People on the Go!, by Zonya Foco

Martha Stewart's Healthy Quick Cook: Four Seasons of Great Menus to Make Everyday Food, by Martha Stewart

Moosewood Restaurant Farm Fresh Meals Deck: 50 Delicious Recipes for Every Season, by the Moosewood Collective

Quick and Healthy Recipes and Ideas: For People Who Say They Don't Have Time to Cook Healthy Meals, 3rd Edition, by Brenda Ponichtera

Quick Flip to Delicious Dinners, by Ellen Faughey

So Easy: Luscious, Healthy Recipes for Every Meal of the Week, by Ellie Krieger

FOOD

Field Guide to Herbs and Spices: How to Identify, Select, and Use Virtually Every Seasoning at the Market, by Aliza Green

Field Guide to Produce: How to Identify, Select, and Prepare Virtually Every Fruit and Vegetable at the Market, by Aliza Green

Food Rules, by Michael Pollan

In Defense of Food, by Michael Pollan

SHARING, SACREDNESS, AND SOULFUL EATING

Care of the Soul, by Thomas Moore

Mindful Eating: A Guide to Rediscovering a Healthy and Joyful Relationship with Food, by Jan Chozen Bays

The Rhythm of Life, by Matthew Kelley

The Sacred Meal: The Ancient Practices Series, by Nora Gallagher

Your Whole Life, by Carol Showalter and Maggie Davis

The Zen of Eating, by Ronna Kabatznick

Recommended Web Resources

www.3DYourWholeLife.com	The 3D program—Your Whole Life
www.BobsRedMill.com	Whole grain products and recipes
www.HodgsonsMill.com	Whole grain products and recipes
www.MyPyramid.gov	USDA Food Pyramid website
www.FoodSafety.gov	U.S. Government Food Safety Website
www.FightBac.org	Partnership for Food Safety Education
www.theWholeGrainCouncil.org	In-depth information on whole grains
www.FoodForLife.com	Ezekiel sprouted organic whole grain products
www.FruitandVeggiesMatter.gov	Centers for Disease Control and Prevention resources
www.SupermarketSavvy.com	Tools to make shopping healthier and easier
www.HarryandDavid.com	Fruit-of-the-Month products
www.Recipes.Sparkpeople.com	Spark People recipes, resources, and community
www.EWG.org/node/27822	Environmental Working Group, Dirty Dozen and Clean Fifteen

Appendix A

T HE FOLLOWING TARGET AMOUNTS of foods are meant to be a proportional guide for planning meals and snacks each day. As you can see, the more calories needed, the greater portions will be from the various core foods and the more choice calories you can consume. This doesn't mean that each day you must consume exactly these amounts. Some days you may be hungrier than on other days.

Above all, consider these targets to aim for, increasing the good foods you plan and consume, while decreasing the less healthy foods that you may have been eating.

Good Food Targets

food group	calories/ serving	800	1000	1200	1400
Vegetables (cups)	25	3	3	4	4
Fruits (cups)	80	2	2	2	2
Whole Grains (1 oz)	80	2	3	3	3
Starches (1 oz)	80	0	0	0	1
High Calcium Foods (1 oz or 1 cup)	100	1.5	1.5	2	2
High Protein Foods (1 oz or 1 cup)	35–75	4	4	5	6
Oils & Other Fats	50	1	2	3	4
Water (8 oz)	0	5	5	6	6

Core Food Calories		750	900	1050	1250
Your Choice Calories		50	100	150	150
Total Calories		800	1000	1200	1400

1600	1800	2000	2200	2400	2600	2800	3000
5	6	6	6	7	7	8	8
3	3	3	3	3	3	4	4
3	3	4	4	5	5	6	6
2	2	3	4	4	5	5	6
2	3	3	3	3	3	3	3
6	6	6	7	7	7	8	8
5	5	6	7	7	8	9	10
7	7	8	8	9	9	10	10

1450	1650	1825	2000	2100	2300	2450	2600
150	150	175	200	300	300	350	400
2600	1800	2000	2200	2400	2600	2800	3000

Food Groups SERVING SIZE COMPARISONS

T HE FOLLOWING SERVING SIZES of different groups of foods are offered for comparison purposes. The portions listed in each food group offer approximately the same amount of calories and carbohydrates. However, they are not the recommended portion for all individuals. They can be useful in determining if you are consuming enough of a specific food to count as a serving. For example, if you are eating an apple that weighs 8 ounces, it would count as 2 servings as listed in the portion guidelines for 1600 Calories. And if you are having ¼ cup of blackberries on your cereal, 1 clementine for a morning snack, and 1 tablespoon of dried cranberries on your salad at lunch, together they would count as a single serving of fruit for the day even though you ate fruit three times that day.

The fruits and vegetables in the following list are marked with asterisks if they are good sources of vitamins C and A, but other deep-colored fruits and vegetables contain smaller amounts of these vitamins, and they can add important nutrients and antioxidants to your daily meals.

Quick Tip Weigh fresh fruits in the store to discover the portion size in ounces.

Fruits (portion sizes vary with the specific fruit)

Apple	4 ounces by weight (1 small apple)
Apricots	4 fresh (5.5 ounces), 4 dried (8 halves)
Banana	½ medium (4 ounces)
Blackberries	¾ cup
Blueberries	¾ cup
Canned fruit	½ cup drained
(including applesauce, apricots, peaches, pears, pineapple, plums, or mixed fruit)	
Cantaloupe*	1 cup cubed
Cherries	12 (3 ounces)

Foods that are good sources of vitamin C   **Foods that are good sources of vitamin A*

▓ Clementines*	2 small (8 ounces)	▓ Mango	½ fruit (5.5 ounces) or ½ cup cubed
▓ Cranberries, dried	2 tablespoons	▓ Nectarine	1 small (5 ounces)
▓ Currants	2 tablespoons	▓ Orange*	1 small (6½ ounces)
▓ Dates	3	▓ Papaya*	½ fruit (8 ounces) or 1 cup cubed
▓ Figs, dried	3 small (1 ounce)	▓ Peach	1 medium (6 ounces)
▓ Figs, fresh	2 medium (3½ ounces)	▓ Pear	1 small or ½ large (4 ounces)
▓ Grapefruit, whole*	½ (11 ounces)	▓ Pineapple	¾ cup cubed
▓ Grapefruit sections*	¾ cup	▓ Plums	2 small (5 ounces)
▓ Grapes	15 (3 ounces)	▓ Pomegranate	½ small (2¾ ounces)
▓ Guava*	1 cup cubed	▓ Raspberries	1 cup
▓ Honeydew	1 cup cubed	▓ Strawberries*	1 cup sliced
▓ Kiwi*	1 (3½ ounces)	▓ Tangerine*	2 small (8 ounces)
▓ Mandarin oranges*	¾ cup	▓ Watermelon	1 cup cubed

Vegetables (1 cup raw or ½ cup cooked or canned provides a serving)

Since the vegetables listed here are very low in calories and provide lots of fiber and nutrients, these portions are designed to help you include a minimum each day according to your meal plan. Consuming more is encouraged!

▓ Artichoke	▓ Carrots**	▓ Hearts of palm
▓ Artichoke hearts	▓ Cauliflower	▓ Jicama
▓ Arugula	▓ Celery	▓ Kale**
▓ Asparagus	▓ Chayote	▓ Kohlrabi
▓ Baby corn	▓ Chicory	▓ Leeks
▓ Bamboo shoots	▓ Collard greens**	▓ Lettuce
▓ Bean sprouts	▓ Cucumber	▓ Mung bean sprouts
▓ Beans, green, wax, or Italian	▓ Eggplant	▓ Mushrooms, all varieties
▓ Beets	▓ Endive	▓ Mustard greens**
▓ Bok choy	▓ Escarole	▓ Okra
▓ Broccoli*	▓ Garlic	▓ Onions
▓ Brussels sprouts*	▓ Green onions	▓ Peppers, all varieties and colors*
▓ Cabbage, all types	▓ Green peas	▓ Radicchio

▓ Radishes, all varieties

▓ Rutabaga

▓ Seaweed

▓ Shallots

▓ Snow peas

▓ Spinach**

▓ Sugar snap peas

▓ Summer squash

▓ Swiss chard**

▓ Tomato

▓ Turnips

▓ Water chestnuts

▓ Watercress

▓ Zucchini

Whole Grains and Cereals

Aim for half your grains to be whole grains, but you could choose all whole grains to add even more fiber and other nutrients to your meals.

▓ Amaranth grain, dry	2 tablespoons
▓ Barley, cooked	⅓ cup
▓ Brown or wild rice, cooked	⅓ cup
▓ Buckwheat flour	3 tablespoons
▓ Buckwheat groats, dry	2 tablespoons
▓ Bulgur wheat, cooked	½ cup
▓ Couscous, cooked, whole-wheat	⅓ cup
▓ Kamut grain, dry	2 tablespoons
▓ Kasha, cooked	½ cup
▓ Quinoa, cooked	⅓ cup
▓ Millet, cooked	⅓ cup
▓ Pasta, whole-grain, cooked	⅓ cup
▓ Polenta, cooked	⅓ cup
▓ Popcorn, air popped, plain	3 cups
▓ Pretzels or baked snack chips	¾ ounce
▓ Oat bran breads (1½ ounces)	1 slice
▓ Triscuit crackers, original or low fat	5
▓ Whole-grain breads, all varieties	1 slice (1 ounce)
▓ Whole-grain sprouted breads	1 slice (1 ounce)

Whole-grain flours, uncooked	3 tablespoons
Whole-grain crackers (includes Kavli, Akmak, Wasa, Finn Crisp, Ryvita)	2

WHOLE-GRAIN CEREALS

Granola, low-fat, low-sugar	¼ cup
Oat bran, dry	¼ cup
Oatmeal, cooked plain	½ cup
Ready-to-eat cereals labeled "Whole Grain"	portion varies
Wheat bran, dry	½ cup
Wheat germ, dry	3 tablespoons

Starches and Starchy Vegetables

NON-WHOLE-GRAIN BREAD PRODUCTS

Bagels	¼ large (1 ounce)
Bread, regular (includes white, multigrain, pumpernickel, rye, and plain raisin bread)	1 slice (1ounce)
Bread, thin-sliced or low-calorie	2 slices (1½ ounces)
Chapatti (6-inch)	1
English muffin	½
Hot dog or burger bun	½ (1 ounce)
Matzoh crackers	¾ ounce
Naan bread (8-inch)	¼
Pancake (4-inch)	1
Pita bread (6-inch)	½
Rice Cakes (4-inch)	2
Roll, medium	½ (2 ounces)

- Tortilla, corn or flour (6-inch) 1
- Waffle (4-inch square)   1

STARCHES (REFINED)

- Breakfast cereals,   ¾ cup
  unsweetened
- Couscous, cooked   ⅓ cup
- Grits, cooked   ½ cup
- Pasta, cooked   ⅓ to ½ cup
- White rice, cooked   ⅓ cup

STARCHY VEGETABLES

- Cassava   ⅓ cup
- Corn kernels, cooked   ½ cup
- Corn on the cob, large ear   ½ cob (5 ounces)
- Hominy   ¾ cup
- Parsnips   ½ cup
- Peas   ½ cup
- Plantain   ⅓ cup
- Potato (white or sweet),   ¼ large potato
  baked with skin   (3 ounces)
- Potato (white or sweet)   ½ cup
  boiled
- Potato (white or sweet),   ½ cup
  mashed plain
- Pumpkin,   1 cup
  canned plain
- Tomato sauce,   ⅓ cup
  canned or jarred
- Winter squash   1 cup
  (butternut, acorn, etc.)**
- Yam, cooked**   ½ cup

Beans, Peas, and Lentils

These versatile foods are also high in protein and fiber. These cooked legumes (½-cup portions) can be counted as 1 starch plus 1 protein.

- Black beans
- Garbanzo beans
  (also known as chickpeas or ceci beans)
- Kidney beans, all colors
- Cannellini beans
- Lima beans
- Navy beans
- Pinto beans
- Fat-free refried beans
- White beans
- Lentils, all colors
- Black-eyed peas
- Split peas
- Baked beans
  (Portion is ⅓ cup because of the calories added by sweet sauce. These have added sugars so the portion is smaller than other types of beans. Use a slotted spoon to drain off some of the sugary sauce.)

High-Calcium Food Sources

Choose nonfat or low-fat whenever possible. I've included the calories as well as the calcium content of these foods since they vary so widely.

	Portion	mg Calcium	Calories
Acidophilus milk or kefir, plain, low-fat	1 cup	250	110
Almond milk, unsweetened	1 cup	200	90
Buttermilk, nonfat	1 cup	250	98
Evaporated skim milk, undiluted	½ cup	370	100
Goat's milk	1 cup	327	168

	Portion	mg Calcium	Calories
Lactaid, skim/nonfat	1 cup	305	80
Rice milk, plain, low-fat	1 cup	300	130
Skim or nonfat milk	1 cup	306	83
Soy milk, light, with added calcium	1 cup	301	80
Soy milk, light, chocolate	1 cup	300	130
Mozzarella cheese, low-fat, shredded	¼ cup	400	70
Cheese, 50% less fat, cheddar	1 ounce	200	70
Yogurt, light	⅔ cup (6 ounces)	200	100
Yogurt, nonfat plain	⅔ cup (6 ounce)	200	75
Collard greens, boiled, drained	⅔ cup	358	61
Spinach, frozen, cooked, drained	1 cup	290	65
Turnip greens, cooked, drained	1 cup	197	29
Orange juice, calcium-fortified	1 cup	266	120

OTHER CALCIUM SOURCES

	Portion	mg Calcium	Calories
Ricotta, part-skim	⅓ cup	132	92
Cottage cheese, low-fat 1%	½ cup	69	81
Yogurt, nonfat Greek style, plain	⅔ cup (6 ounce)	112	90
Yogurt, nonfat Greek style w/honey	⅔ cup (6 ounce)	91	204
Yogurt, frozen, low-fat, vanilla	½ cup	100	140
Ice cream, vanilla, not premium	½ cup	80	150
Chocolate pudding, no sugar added	½ cup	40	60
N.E. Clam chowder, 98% fat-free	1 cup	20	105
Pinto beans, canned	1 cup	80	220
Bok choy	1 cup	160	20
Kale, frozen, boiled	1 cup	180	39
Mustard greens, frozen, cooked, drained	1 cup	152	28
Swiss chard, cooked, drained	1 cup	101	35

CALCIUM SUPPLEMENTS

Choose another food, such as 1 ounce of lean meat or a fruit, to replace the calories and protein of dairy foods.

	Portion	mg Calcium	Calories
Adora calcium, dark chocolate	1 piece	500	30
Viactiv calcium chews	1 piece	400	20
Calcium citrate, tablet or gel cap	1	300–600	0

Lean High-Protein Foods

When planning portions, generally 4 ounces of raw meat, fish, or poultry will yield 3 ounces cooked, or a 75% cooked yield; the leaner and lower in fat the food, the less loss in cooking. The leaner the protein, the less saturated (unhealthy) fat, so be sure to look for lean cuts and trim off visible fat before cooking.

FISH (1 ounce cooked)

- Anchovies, catfish, cod, flounder, haddock, halibut, herring, lox (smoked salmon), mahi mahi, monkfish, orange roughy, salmon, sardines, sole, swordfish, tilapia, trout, tuna

SHELLFISH AND CRUSTACEANS (1 ounce cooked)

- Clams, crab, imitation crab or shellfish, langoustines, lobster, mussels, oysters (6 count as 1 ounce), scallops, shrimp

MEAT (1 ounce cooked)

- Beef trimmed of visible fat: chuck, rib, rump, round, sirloin, tenderloin
- Lean ground beef 85% or more lean; the higher the percentage of lean, the lower the fat and calories.
- Lamb chops, leg of lamb, lamb roasts, lean ground lamb
- Pork loin, rib chop, or roast, tenderloin, lean cutlets, lean ground pork
- Sausage containing 3 grams or less of fat per ounce
- Veal loin, tenderloin, lean cutlets, lean ground veal

POULTRY (1 ounce cooked)
- Skinless chicken, Cornish hen, turkey

EGGS (1 ounce)
- Whole eggs (1), egg whites (1)
- Egg substitutes (¼ cup)

CHEESE AND YOGURT
- Hard and Soft Cheeses with 3 grams or less fat per ounce, soy cheese, rice cheese (1 ounce)
- Cottage Cheese (¼ cup for 1 ounce protein)
- Greek Nonfat Yogurt ($\frac{1}{3}$ cup for 1 ounce protein)
- Regular Plain Yogurt (1 cup for 1 ounce protein)

Plant-based proteins

These may contain lean protein plus a carbohydrate or fat serving; check the package label to evaluate the ingredients and the nutrient content.

BEANS AND LENTILS
- All except baked beans (½ cup for 1 ounce protein and 1 starch)
- Baked Beans ($\frac{1}{3}$ cup for 1 ounce protein and 1 starch)

NUTS
- Peanut butter (2 tablespoons for 1 protein and 1 fat)
- Soy nuts (¼ cup for 1 protein)

SOY
- Tofu (½ cup for 1 ounce protein)
- Tempeh (¼ cup for 1 ounce protein and 1 fat)
- Edamame, green soy beans (½ cup for 1 ounce protein and ½ starch)

MEAT SUBSTITUTES
- Quorn (mycoprotein) plain cutlet (1 ounce protein)
- Quorn (mycoprotein) chicken-style patty (1 ounce protein, 1 fat, and 1 starch)

■ Soy meat patties, sausages, or "crumbles" (2 ounces for 1 protein and ½ starch)

■ Soy sausage patties or links (1½ ounces for 1 protein and 1 fat)

■ Near East falafel mix (⅓ cup uncooked for 1 protein and 1 starch)

Healthy Fats and Oils

The healthiest fats are generally found in plant-based foods. These foods contain significant amounts of monounsaturated fats. But some processed oils change chemically to more closely resemble saturated (unhealthy) animal fats. One example would be vegetable shortening, which is solid at room temperature.

OILS

■ from olives, avocado, canola, coconut, corn,   1 teaspoon oil
grape seed, hazelnut, peanut, sesame seeds,
soybean, walnut

NUTS

(number of whole nuts that provides 1 healthy fat serving)

■ Almonds	6
■ Brazil nuts	2
■ Cashews	5
■ Hazelnuts	5
■ Macadamias	2
■ Peanuts	20
■ Pecan halves	3
■ Pine nuts	1 tablespoon
■ Pistachios	14
■ Soy nuts	1 tablespoon
■ Walnut halves	4

OLIVES

Kalamata	5
Manzanilla, green, stuffed	6
Jumbo black	7
Green, small	10
Small black	12

AVOCADO (⅛ whole avocado or 2 tablespoons for 1 fat)

SEEDS

Flaxseed, whole or ground	1 tablespoon
Pumpkin, sunflower, sesame	1 tablespoon
Tahini (sesame paste)	2 teaspoons

SALAD DRESSINGS made with olive oil, light   2 tablespoons

SALAD DRESSINGS made with olive oil, regular   1 tablespoon

Other less healthy fats

Limit your intake of these fats, which are high in saturated and polyunsaturated fats. Choose healthier fats whenever you can.

Margarine, low-fat, light	1 tablespoon
Margarine, stick or tub	1 teaspoon
Mayonnaise, reduced-fat	1 tablespoon
Mayonnaise, regular	2 teaspoons
Salad dressings, reduced-fat	2 tablespoons
Salad dressings, regular	2 teaspoons

SATURATED FATS

- Bacon   1 slice
- Butter, stick   1 teaspoon
- Butter, whipped   2 teaspoons
- Coconut, shredded   2 tablespoons
- Coconut milk, light   ⅓ cup
- Coconut milk, regular   1½ tablespoons
- Cream, half-and-half   2 tablespoons
- Cream, light   1½ tablespoons
- Cream, heavy, liquid   1 tablespoon
- Cream, heavy, whipped   2 tablespoons
- Cream, whipped in can   3 tablespoons (¼ cup)
- Cream cheese, reduced fat   1½ tablespoons
- Cream cheese, regular   1 tablespoon
- Oil, coconut, palm   1 teaspoon
- Lard   1 teaspoon
- Solid vegetable shortening   1 teaspoon
- Sour cream, light   3 tablespoons
- Sour cream, regular   2 tablespoons

Acknowledgments

FIRST, I WOULD LIKE TO THANK my husband, Steve, and my daughter, Eleanor, who have shared my life and my table and have endured my constant experimentation in the kitchen. And thanks to my friends who have happily broken bread with me through good times and bad. Special thanks go to all of my clients, patients, and colleagues who have taught me so much about food and life.

I am grateful to my editors Jon Sweeney, Lil Copan, and Bob Edmonson, and to the staff at Paraclete Press for their patience and guidance on translating my philosophy and expertise into book form.

And special thanks to Carol Showalter, my co-author of *Your Whole Life*, and the best role model I know for living a whole life.

Index

The 3D Prayer

Dear Lord,
This is a new day
That means I can expect from your hand
    all I need to live.
Help me to know
Your grace is sufficient
Your power is overwhelming
    and your peace and joy are here for the asking.
I need you in so many practical ways, Lord
I need you to help me choose the right spirit
    at the beginning of the day
I need you to help me with my family
    the work I need to get done
    and the pressures that come at me
    before my eyes are even open.
I need you to go ahead of me every step of the way
You will do that
This day is yours
I am yours.
Thank you for loving me and giving me
    the gift of life today.
When I am ready to close my eyes
    at the end of this day
May I say with a steady voice:
I have loved you more today than I did yesterday
But not as much as I will tomorrow.
Make it so, dear Lord.
Amen.

The foundational Book and Journal.
It all begins here.

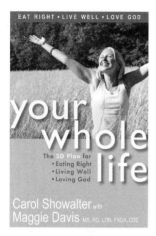

Your Whole Life

This is the latest edition of the book that has taken millions of people on the journey to health and wholeness. Carol Showalter and Maggie Davis guide you for the first twelve weeks in making small, gradual, positive changes that are proven to become permanent. Ideal for group use, *Your Whole Life* includes easy-to-navigate nutritional goals and advice, abundant tips for living well, and daily Bible readings and inspiration.

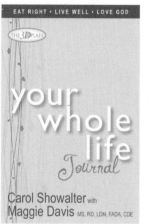

Your Whole Life JOURNAL

Record your progress with this convenient, inspirational, spiral-bound Journal, designed to be your close companion for the first twelve weeks. You'll find that you turn to it like a friend.

Includes:

- A message from Your Whole Life founder, Carol Showalter
- Daily nutritional guides and reminders
- Inspirational Bible verses and other inspirations
- Space for your own note-taking and spiritual reflections

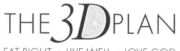

THE 3D PLAN

EAT RIGHT · LIVE WELL · LOVE GOD

For more information, and for additional resources, go to www.3DYourWholeLife.com
or call and speak with us at 1-800-451-5006.